OXFORD ASSESS AND PROGRESS

Series Editors

Katharine Boursicot
Director, Health Professional Assessment Consultancy (HPAC)
Honorary Reader in Medical Education, St George's,
University of London

David Sales
Consultant in Medical Asse~

D0534144

OXFORD ASSESS AND PROGRESS
your prescription for exam success

Written by clinicians and educational experts, these unique guides present complete coverage for your exam revision, with illustrative material and tips to help you succeed in your medical exams.

Also available and forthcoming titles in the Oxford Assess and Progress series

Clinical Medicine, Second Edition
Alex Liakos and Martin Hill

Clinical Specialties, Third Edition
Luci Etheridge and Alex Bonner

Clinical Surgery
Neil Borley, Frank Smith, Paul McGovern, Bernadette Pereira, and Oliver Old

Emergency Medicine
Pawan Gupta

Medical Sciences
Jade Chow and John Patterson

Psychiatry
Gil Myers and Melissa Gardner

OXFORD ASSESS AND PROGRESS

Situational Judgement Test

Third Edition

David Metcalfe
University of Oxford

Harveer Dev
University of Cambridge

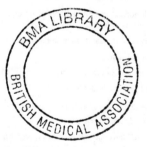

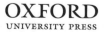

OXFORD
UNIVERSITY PRESS

OXFORD
UNIVERSITY PRESS

Great Clarendon Street, Oxford, OX2 6DP,
United Kingdom

Oxford University Press is a department of the University of Oxford.
It furthers the University's objective of excellence in research, scholarship,
and education by publishing worldwide. Oxford is a registered trade mark of
Oxford University Press in the UK and in certain other countries

First Edition published in 2012
Second Edition published in 2014
Third Edition published in 2018

Impression: 2

Published in the United States of America by Oxford University Press
198 Madison Avenue, New York, NY 10016, United States of America

British Library Cataloguing in Publication Data

Data available

Library of Congress Control Number: 2017956889

ISBN 978–0–19–880580–9

Printed and bound in Great Britain by
Ashford Colour Press Ltd.

Oxford University Press makes no representation, express or implied, that the
drug dosages in this book are correct. Readers must therefore always check
the product information and clinical procedures with the most up-to-date
published product information and data sheets provided by the manufacturers
and the most recent codes of conduct and safety regulations. The authors and
the publishers do not accept responsibility or legal liability for any errors in the
text or for the misuse or misapplication of material in this work. Except where
otherwise stated, drug dosages and recommendations are for the non-pregnant
adult who is not breast-feeding

Foreword

Being a doctor is a huge privilege—we touch and change lives and enjoy unparalleled levels of public trust. But the high reputation enjoyed by the medical profession depends on all who practise medicine behaving in a way that continues to command confidence and respect. A great deal of what we do depends on knowledge and skills, and we all keep learning new facts or embracing new ideas throughout our careers. But there is another and equally important aspect of being a doctor and that is about knowing our limitations. Really good doctors will know the limit of what they know and what they can do. No one—most of all the patient you're seeing at that moment—will thank you for doing something that you're simply not able to do. Whether it's thinking that you remember the dose of a drug but not checking, or soldiering on because you think it's a sign of weakness to ask for help, or advising someone about the risks of a procedure you've never done, or myriad other pitfalls, knowing the limits of your own abilities is one of a doctor's most important qualities.

The General Medical Council has been guiding doctors in the area of professionalism for over 150 years. The world has changed a lot over that time, but some of the qualities that define the physician are timeless and have endured. This book guides you through various scenarios where your professionalism could be tested and helpfully references some of our guidance. The message is simple but fundamentally important: saying that you don't know, but will find someone who does, is a sign of professional maturity.

Professor Sir Peter Rubin
Former Chair, (2009–2015), General Medical Council

Series editor preface

The Oxford Assess and Progress series started as a groundbreaking development in the extensive area of self-assessment texts available for medical studies. The majority of volumes are linked to the Oxford Handbook series, with specially commissioned modern-format questions constructed to test the problem-solving skills used by practising clinicians in order to deliver high-quality and safe patient care by recognizing, understanding, and treating common problems, as well as recognizing less likely, but potentially catastrophic, conditions.

With the increasing emphasis on the professionalism of doctors, and the requirement to test and demonstrate professional values and behaviour, a new format of questions has been developed and introduced into selection procedures for a number of postgraduate education and training circumstances. These questions are known collectively as a Situational Judgement Test (SJT), which is designed to test certain attributes deemed to be desirable in practising medical professionals, encompassing the values, attitudes, and behaviours expected of new doctors as set out in the General Medical Council's documents *Good Medical Practice* (2013) and *Tomorrow's Doctors* (2009).

This particular volume is special as it is written for this new question format, but in keeping with the rest of the series, it has a number of unique features and is designed as much as a formative learning resource as a self-assessment one. The current position of the SJT within the selection to the Foundation Programme in the UK is explained in detail, with advice on how to approach this new set of tests.

The test items place the candidate in professionally challenging situations, and a number of possible reactions are offered. Attention has been paid to explaining learning points and constructive feedback on each question, using clear fact- or evidence-based explanations as to why the 'correct' response is the most appropriate and why the other responses are less appropriate. This is especially important as SJTs require consideration of the most appropriate responses to a given professional dilemma, where no single answer is completely correct or incorrect.

As the use of SJTs is likely to expand into more contexts where doctors' professionalism, values, and attitudes will be formally tested, this volume is a leading-edge introduction on how to prepare for the future of such testing.

Katharine Boursicot

Author preface

With finals on the horizon, you might be tempted to coast through the Situational Judgement Test (SJT). The Foundation Programme is *generic* as all trainees develop the same core skills and competencies, and you might be told that your choice of FY1/FY2 rotations 'doesn't really matter'.

The truth is that your clinical rotations might easily shape the rest of your career. It's unsurprising that most doctors settle in the area to which they are allocated for their first job. But your rotations are also important for progressing to the next stage of your chosen specialty. Although specific clinical experience is never mandatory, it is easier to argue convincingly that you want to work in a specialty if you have relevant audit projects, contacts, and experience. The best way to develop a specialty-specific portfolio is to secure your first-choice rotation. If you have strong feelings about where you want to work or your future specialty, you need to maximize your SJT score.

You might also hear that you 'can't study' for the SJT. We have sat many exams between us and have yet to come across one that can't be beaten with hard work and adequate preparation.

This book will help you become familiar with the style and content of SJT questions. Practice questions and familiarity with professional guidance are vital to maximizing your SJT score.

Best of luck with the SJT and securing your first-choice rotation!

David Metcalfe
Harveer Dev

Acknowledgements

It would not have been possible to produce this book without the help of many individuals and their institutions. In particular:

All the reviewers (p. xix–p. xx) who helped to produce thought-pro-voking questions and carefully considered explanations.

The invaluable principles laid out by the General Medical Council (p. 20) on which our answers are based. In particular, we must thank Professor Sir Peter Rubin for contributing the foreword.

Our editorial team at Oxford University Press, specifically Fiona Richardson, Hannah Lloyd, Geraldine Jeffers, and series editor Katharine Boursicot.

Mina, Jasvinder, and Bobby for their continued support for, and patience with, the editors.

Acknowledgements

Contents

Series editors

Professor Katharine Boursicot BSc MBBS MRCOG MAHPE NTF SFHEA FRSM is a consultant in health professions education, with special expertise in assessment. Previously she was Head of Assessment at St George's, University of London, Barts, and the London School of Medicine and Dentistry, and Associate Dean for Assessment at Cambridge University School of Clinical Medicine. She is consultant on assessment to several UK medical schools, medical Royal Colleges, and international institutions, as well as an assessment advisor to the General Medical Council.

David Sales is a general practitioner by training who has been involved in medical assessment for over 20 years, having previously been convenor of the MRCGP knowledge test. He has run item-writing workshops for a number of undergraduate medical schools and medical Royal Colleges, and internationally. He currently chairs the Professional and Linguistic Assessments Board Part 1 panel for the General Medical Council, and is their consultant on Fitness to Practise knowledge testing.

About the authors

David Metcalfe holds first class honours degrees in Biological Sciences with Molecular Genetics (BSc) and Law (LLB). He graduated with an MB ChB from Warwick Medical School in 2010. He is currently a Clinical Research Fellow in Musculoskeletal Trauma at the University of Oxford and Specialty Registrar in Trauma and Orthopaedic Surgery within the West Midlands Deanery. He has previously taught ethics and medical law at University College London.

Harveer Dev graduated with a BA(Hons) in Natural Sciences (2008) and an MB BChir (2011) from the University of Cambridge. He is an NIHR Academic Clinical Fellow in Urology at Addenbrooke's Hospital in Cambridge. He studied the role of DNA repair in cancer as a Fulbright Scholar at Harvard University and is continuing this work as part of a Wellcome Trust PhD Fellowship at the University of Cambridge. He currently serves as a magistrate for the Central London Bench.

Reviewers

Laura Barnfield MBChB
DRCOG DGM MRCGP
Greater Manchester, UK

Elizabeth Bird-Lieberman
MA PhD MRCP
University of Cambridge,
Cambridge, UK

Daniel Border
BSc(Hons) MBChB
University Hospital Coventry &
Warwickshire, Coventry, UK

James Chambers BSc(Hons)
MBChB MRCS FRCR
Mersey School of Radiology,
Liverpool, UK

Dan Cooper BSc(Hons) MRCP
Royal Liverpool University
Hospital, Liverpool, UK

Susie Cooper
MBChB MRCPCH
Princess Ann Hospital,
Southampton, UK

William Coppola BMBCh MA
DRCOG MRCGP
University College London
Medical School, London, UK

Harveer Dev MA MRCS
Addenbrooke's Hospital,
Cambridge, UK

Jon Downing
BSc(Hons) MBChB
Great Western Hospital,
Swindon, UK

Oghenekome Gbinigie
MA(Cantab) MB BChir MRCGP
DRCOG DfSRH
University College Hospital,
London, UK

John Gomes MBBS PhD MRCP
London, UK

Ruth Green MEng(Hons)
MA MBBS
St George's Hospital, London, UK

Alison Ho MA MBBS
St Peter's Hospital, Chertsey, UK

Kulvir Hundal BSc(Hons)
MBChB MRCGP
Birmingham, UK

Tariq Husain BSc(Hons) MA
MRCP FRCA DICM
Northwick Park Hospital,
Harrow, UK

Syed Jafery MBBS
Queen Elizabeth Hospital, King's
Lynn, UK

Reena Johal MBChB
MRCP MRCGP
Birmingham, UK

Vasha Kaur
MBChB(Hons) FRCS
London, UK

Jayne Kavanagh BA(Hons)
MA MBChB
University College London,
London, UK

Hugh Mackenzie
BSc(Hons) MRCS
St Mary's Hospital,
London, UK

David McKean MA BMBCh
John Radcliffe Hospital,
Oxford, UK

Eleanor Mearing-Smith
BSc(Hons) MRCS
London, UK

David Metcalfe LLB(Hons)
MRCP MRCS
University of Oxford, UK

Fiona Molloy
BSc(Hons) MBChB
Royal Victoria Hospital, Ireland

Gabriella Muallem
BSc(Hons) MBBS
Royal Surrey County Hospital,
Guildford, UK

Lindsay Muscroft
BSc(Hons) MBChB
University Hospitals Leicester,
Leicester, UK

Georgina Naidoo MBChB
Preston, Lancashire, UK

Vinnie Nambisan BSc(Hons)
MA MRCP
Saint Francis Hospice,
Romford, UK

Katherine Oliver BMedSci
MBBCh MRCGP
London, UK

Janso Padickakudi MBBCh
MSc MRCS
East of England Deanery, UK

Vinod Patel BSc(Hons) MD
FRCP MRCGP DRCOG FHEA
George Eliot Hospital,
Nuneaton, UK

Bilal Salman
BSc(Hons) MBChB
Warwick Hospital,
Warwickshire, UK

Stephan Sanders
BMedSci(Hons) BMBS PhD
University of California, San
Francisco, California, USA

Clare Smith BSc(Hons)
MBChB MRCGP
Oxford, UK

Prasanna Sooriakumaran
PhD FRCS(Urol)
University College London
Hospital, London, UK

Abhishek Srivastava MD
Albert Einstein College of
Medicine, New York, USA

Kapil Sugand BSc(Hons)
MBBS MRCS
North West London, UK

Yew-Wei Tan MBChB MRCS
Addenbrooke's Hospital,
Cambridge, UK

Jason Thompson BSc(Hons)
MBChB PhD
Royal Sussex County Hospital,
Brighton, UK

Thomas Troth MBChB
Birmingham, UK

Daniel Westacott
FRCS(Orth)
University Hospitals Coventry
& Warwickshire NHS Trust,
Coventry, UK

Tom Whitfield BMBS
Royal Adelaide Hospital,
Adelaide, Australia

Siobhan Wild BMBS
St George's Hospital, London, UK

Timothy Williamson
BSc(Hons) MBChB
University of East Anglia,
Norwich, UK

Explanation of terms

Most of the terms used in these questions should be familiar, but you should note the following.

Clinical Supervisor

The person directly responsible for your day-to-day clinical practice. This will almost always be one of the consultants leading your team. You should approach them about problems with the team, post, or patients under their care.

Educational Supervisor

The person responsible for your professional development through a number of rotations (e.g. the whole of FY1). They have a more global view of your progress and ensure continuity as you move between posts. You should approach them about career plans, pastoral concerns, and problems with your Clinical Supervisor.

Clinical Director

The senior clinician (usually a consultant) with responsibility for a particular department within a hospital, e.g. the Emergency Department.

Medical Director

A senior doctor (i.e. a consultant) with management responsibilities at a trust level. The Medical Director is generally more senior than the Clinical Directors.

A&E	Accident and Emergency
ABG	Arterial Blood Gas
ALS	Advanced Life Support
AMTS	Abbreviated Mental Test Score
ATLS	Advanced Trauma Life Support
BMA	British Medical Association
BMI	Body Mass Index
CAGE	Concern, Anger, Guilt, Eye opener
CCG	Clinical Commissioning Group
COPD	Chronic Obstructive Pulmonary Disease
CT	Computed Tomography (scan)
CTPA	Computed Tomography Pulmonary Angiography
DNACPR	Do Not Attempt Cardio-Pulmonary Resuscitation
DVLA	Driver and Vehicle Licensing Agency

EPM	Educational Performance Measure
FACD	Foundation Achievement of Competence Document
FY1	Foundation Year 1 (doctor)
FY2	Foundation Year 2 (doctor)
GCS	Glasgow Coma Scale
GP	General Practice
GMC	General Medical Council
HCA	Healthcare Assistant
HIV	Human Immunodeficiency Virus
HPA	Health Protection Agency
HR	Human Resources
ISFP	Improving Selection to the Foundation Programme
ITU	Intensive Therapy Unit
KUB	Kidney–Ureter–Bladder
MAU	Medical Admissions Unit
MDT	Multi-Disciplinary Team
MPS	Medical Protection Society
MRI	Magnetic Resonance Imaging
NSAID	Non-Steroidal Anti-Inflammatory Drug
OGD	Oesophagogastroduodenoscopy
PALS	Patient Advice and Liaison Service
PPH	Postpartum Haemorrhage
PPI	Proton Pump Inhibitor
PRN	As Required
RCP	Royal College of Physicians
SHO	Senior House Officer
SJT	Situational Judgement Test
TAB	Team Assessment of Behaviour
TB	Tuberculosis
UKCAT	UK Clinical Aptitude Test
UKFPO	UK Foundation Programme Office

Section 1

Introduction to the SJT

Chapter 1

Foundation Programme selection

New doctors intending to work in the United Kingdom (UK) should complete the Foundation Programme. This two-year schedule of rotations ensures core competencies are achieved before doctors enter further training.

The first foundation year (FY1) is intended for medical graduates to begin taking supervised responsibility for patient care. Completion of FY1 will usually lead to full registration with the General Medical Council (GMC) and automatic progression to a further year of training. Doctors take on additional responsibility in the second foundation year (FY2) and its successful completion results in the award of a Foundation Achievement of Competence Document (FACD). The FACD indicates that a doctor has achieved the competences necessary to begin one of the many core or specialty training programmes.

Selection to the Foundation Programme is overseen by the UK Foundation Programme Office (UKFPO). This organization is responsible for allocating final-year medical students to their new foundation schools.

Allocation of posts

Allocation to foundation schools depends on a score achieved by each student. Applicants through the UKFPO must rank all foundation schools (Units of Application) during the online application process.

The system begins with the highest-scoring applicant and assigns them their first-choice foundation school. It does the same for the second highest-scoring applicant and continues in this vein. Once the system reaches an applicant whose first-choice foundation school is 'full', they are assigned their second choice, and so on.

Therefore, the key determinants as to whether an applicant is placed in their first-choice location are their UKFPO 'score' and the popularity of their chosen foundation school. The ratio of first-choice applicants to places varies every year, but some foundation schools (e.g. Oxford and those in London) are almost always oversubscribed.

Therefore, it is important to understand how scores are assigned and maximize your performance on these measures.

Assignment of scores

Until 2012 entry, student preferences were allocated according to two measures:

1. Position within their medical school cohort by quartile. Quartiles were determined locally by each medical school with only general guidance from the UKFPO.
2. Answers provided on an application form which asked about academic achievements but weighted most points towards short essay-type answers.

This system was widely perceived as stressful and unfair by students. Such concerns led to a project called Improving Selection to the Foundation Programme (ISFP). After a wide-ranging review, ISFP proposed a revised system to distinguish between new doctors. In brief, this also includes two components:

1. Educational Performance Measure (EPM).
2. Situational Judgement Test (SJT).

Educational Performance Measure

The EPM is an attempt at measuring academic performance. It comprises three parts:

1. Medical school performance (34–43 points).
2. Degrees (0–5).
3. Publications (0–2).

Medical school performance is still determined locally but by deciles to achieve finer discrimination. The assessments counting towards this score and their respective weighting should be (or have been) discussed with your cohort representatives.

The points for academic qualifications are shown in Table 1.1.

Table 1.1 Points awarded for qualifications

Qualification	Points
Doctoral degree	5
Master's degree	4
First-class honours degree* BDS/BVetMed	
2.1 honours degree*	3
2.2 honours degree*	2
Third-class, unclassified, or ordinary honours degree*	1
Primary medical qualification	0

*Intercalated degrees that do not extend the course length (e.g. the BMedSci awarded by the University of Nottingham) are awarded one point less for each honours category.

One point is awarded towards the EPM for each publication you are named on as an author with a PubMed ID—up to a maximum of two points.

Be aware that only five points can be awarded for degrees and two for publications. Therefore, an applicant with both first-class honours and a Master's degree will score four points in the degrees category.

Situational Judgement Test

Your EPM score is difficult to influence if you are within a year of applying to the Foundation Programme.

The good news (for most students) is that the EPM is actually the minority component. Officially, the EPM is out of 50 points and SJT scores are similarly recalibrated to a 50-point scale. However, you may recall that the lowest possible EPM score is 34 points (p. 4). This means there are *only 17* possible points between a student in the bottom decile with no academic achievements and the highest achiever with a PhD and a string of publications.

All applicants should therefore seek to maximize their score on the second component—the SJT. Fortunately you are off to a good start by reading this book!

Chapter 2

What is the SJT?

SJTs are commonly used by organizations for personnel selection. They aim to provide realistic, but hypothetical, scenarios and possible answers which are either selected or ranked by the candidate.

One such test will contribute half, or significantly more than half (p. 5), the score used by applicants to the UK Foundation Programme.

Mechanics of the SJT

The test will involve a single paper over two hours and twenty minutes in which candidates will answer 70 questions. This equates to approximately two minutes per question. Your response to 60 questions will be included in your final score, while ten questions embedded throughout the test will be pilot questions which are designed to be validated but not counted in your final score. You will not be able to differentiate pilot from genuine test questions and should answer every question as if it 'counts'.

In one SJT pilot (p. 18), 96% of candidates finished the test within two hours, which provides some indication about the time pressure. It is important to answer all questions and not simply 'guess' those left at the end. Although the SJT is not negatively marked, random guesses are not allocated points. The scoring software will identify guesses by looking for unusual or sporadic answer patterns.

The SJT will be held locally by individual medical schools under invigilated conditions. Therefore, your medical school should be in touch about specific local arrangements.

Each SJT paper will include a selection of questions, each mapped to a specific professional attribute (p. 11). Questions should be evenly distributed between attributes and between scenario type, i.e. 'patient', 'colleague', or 'personal'.

The SJT will include two types of question:

- multiple choice questions (approximately one-third)
- ranking questions (approximately two-thirds).

Multiple choice questions

These begin with a scenario and provide eight possible answers. Three of these are correct and should be selected. The remaining five are incorrect.

The example in Box 2.1 provides an illustrative medical school scenario. For questions based around Foundation Programme scenarios, over 100 examples are provided for practice from p. 231 onwards.

Box 2.1 An example multiple choice question

All of your friends have received an email from the medical school, allocating a piece of work. You have not received any such correspondence.

Choose the THREE most appropriate actions to take in this situation.

A Ignore the email as it has not been sent to you.

B Write a complaint to the administrator as she has left you off the mailing list.

C Complete the piece of work and submit it by the deadline.

D Ask the administrator if the email was intended for you as well.

E Keep quiet as this will guarantee you an extension.

F Ask your friends for details to assess whether you should have been included.

G Check whether any other important emails have gone astray.

H Use a friend's work as a basis for your own to save time.

The answer in this case might be D, F, G.

Each correct answer scores four marks, and so the highest score for each question is 12. It is important to note that if more than three options are chosen, the whole question is awarded zero.

Ranking questions

Ranking questions begin with a scenario and provide five possible answers. You must rank the answers from 'most appropriate' to 'least appropriate'. This is challenging as it may require you to choose between conflicting values. It might also be difficult to determine which of two *inappropriate* actions is the least appropriate.

A medical school example might be along the lines of that shown in Box 2.2.

Box 2.2 An example ranking question

You arrive ten minutes late for a mandatory lecture. As you peer through the doors, you see there are no spaces on the back row and you will have to disturb a number of settled students to find a seat.

Rank in order the following actions in response to this situation (1 = Most appropriate; 5 = Least appropriate).

A Go to the library and study the lecture material before slipping in for the next session.

B Head into the lecture theatre and move people along the row so that you can get a seat.

C Sign the attendance register and then wait for your friends in the coffee shop.

D Head into the lecture theatre and move a lot of people so you can get to your favourite seat in the middle of a row.

E Go to the coffee shop until the lecture ends and you can slip in for the next session.

The answer in this case might be B, A, E, D, C.

The lecture is mandatory and you should attend, even if this means politely disturbing some of your colleagues (B). Studying the material elsewhere is less ideal, as you are supposed to attend the session (A). However, studying the material is preferable to sitting in the coffee shop (E). Sitting in the coffee shop waiting for the next session might in turn be a better option than disturbing many of your colleagues (and potentially the lecture itself) unnecessarily (D). However, the least appropriate option is signing the attendance register when you have not attended the session (C). This is dishonest and casts considerable doubt on your professional probity.

The scoring of such ranking questions is complicated. Each question is marked out of 20 potential points, as illustrated in Fig. 2.1.

	Applicant order				
Correct order	**1**	**2**	**3**	**4**	**5**
1	4	3	2	1	0
2	3	4	3	2	1
3	2	3	4	3	2
4	1	2	3	4	3
5	0	1	2	3	4

Figure 2.1 A grid for calculating points for ranking question answers

This system means that a complete answer will always score a minimum of 8/20.

Thus, if you had selected A, D, C, B, E in the example described previously, your score would be 10/20, as illustrated in Fig. 2.2.

Correct order	Applicant order				
	A	**D**	**C**	**B**	**E**
B	4	3	2	1	0
A	3	4	3	2	1
E	2	3	4	3	2
C	1	2	3	4	3
D	0	1	2	3	4

Figure 2.2 A worked example grid with 10/20 points scored for the answer ADCBE

It is important to note that if two options are given the same ranking, both tied options will be awarded zero. Tying options is the only way to score less than eight and so is best avoided unless you are feeling particularly experimental!

Chapter 3

What does the SJT test?

The SJT was developed to test nine professional attributes identified from a detailed analysis of the FY1 role. These attributes are as follows:

1. **Commitment to professionalism**
2. **Coping with pressure**
3. **Effective communication**
4. Learning and professional development
5. Organization and planning
6. **Patient focus**
7. Problem-solving and decision-making
8. Self-awareness and insight
9. **Working effectively as part of a team**

However, the SJT recognizes that there is considerable overlap between these attributes and that some cannot be effectively assessed with a written test. As a result, SJT questions focus on the five attributes highlighted in bold.

It is worth considering what the SJT requires of candidates according to each key attribute.

Commitment to professionalism

Candidates must be honest, trustworthy, reliable, and aware of ethical issues (e.g. confidentiality). They should challenge behaviour that is unacceptable or risks patient safety. Candidates should take appropriate responsibility for their own actions and omissions.

Coping with pressure

Candidates must be resilient and remain calm under pressure. Judgement should not be affected by pressure and candidates should develop appropriate coping strategies.

...mmunication

...e (verbally and in writing) concisely and
...vary their communication style appropri-
...willing to engage others in open dialogue.

Patient focus

Candidates should always show respect to patients. They should adopt a collaborative approach to decision-making with patients as well as maintaining courtesy, empathy, and compassion.

Working effectively as part of a team

Candidates should be able to work in partnership while respecting different views. They should share tasks fairly and ask advice from others when necessary.

Should, not *would*, questions

Despite appearances, the SJT is a *knowledge-based* examination. It is important to remember throughout that questions ask what you *should* do, rather than what you *would* do in any given situation. Therefore, it is a test of whether you know the 'correct' action and not whether you would act correctly if working as a doctor.

For example, a question might introduce you as an FY1 doctor on a busy ward. You are told to examine an elderly patient of the opposite sex and all the nurses are occupied elsewhere. You might have seen doctors examine patients under these circumstances without a chaperone. You might even think that this would be your approach in real life. However, you know on some level that a better solution is to insist on (or at least to offer) the presence of a chaperone. Therefore, this option is likely to rank above continuing to examine the patient.

Does it work?

Improving Selection to the Foundation Programme (ISFP) undertook a wide-ranging review of options for allocating new doctors to FY1 posts. It selected the SJT.

Whether the SJT works or not depends on whether it can accurately predict 'good' doctors. There is no real consensus about how to measure the effectiveness of foundation doctors, and so the SJT question is unlikely to ever be resolved to everyone's satisfaction. However, variations on the SJT have been used in selection to some specialties (e.g. general practice (GP) and public health training). They are also used by many firms in the commercial sector.

The SJT pilots suggested a high degree of internal reliability ($\alpha = 0.79$–0.85). It was also shown that SJT performance is positively correlated with extraversion, openness, and achievement. A subsequent study (MacKenzie *et al*. 2017) has shown that SJT score was predicted by emotional non-defensiveness, aloofness, and empathy, as suggested by the non-cognitive component of the UK Clinical Aptitude Test (UKCAT). The SJT score is also correlated with UKFPO performance (MacKenzie *et al*. 2016). Interestingly, SJT score is not correlated with performance at medical school as measured by the EPM (Simon *et al*. 2015).

Advantages of the SJT over the previously used 'white space' questions (p. 4) include the following:

- invigilated conditions so that no one can seek external help with answers
- less reliance on creative writing skills
- questions directly address prioritization, teamworking, and professionalism—all of which are important qualities for new doctors
- evidence from other sectors suggests that situational judgement questions can effectively predict job performance.

Although students are unlikely to relish sitting another high-stakes examination in their final year, earlier selection methods were perceived as both burdensome and unfair. A number of studies have suggested that the SJT is unpopular amongst both medical students and faculty members (Sharma, 2015; Sharma *et al*. 2016). It is impossible to please everyone and you are most likely to approve of this method in retrospect if your score is high enough.

Criticisms of the SJT include:

- As noted on p. 5, the SJT and EPM are not equally weighted. As the latter is essentially scored along a 17-point scale (compared to the 50-point SJT scale), the SJT is weighted almost three times as heavily as the EPM. Many students have objected to their whole medical school experience being marginalized in this way when it comes to applying for jobs.
- There is very little variation from the mean in terms of student performance. The *BMJ Careers* article detailed at the end of this chapter

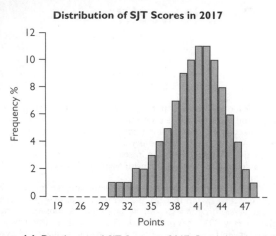

Figure 4.1 Distribution of SJT Scores in 2017. Reproduced with kind permission from the UK Foundation Programme Office http://www.foundationprogramme.nhs.uk/pages/fp-afp/faqs/SJT.

calculated that omitting a single question from the SJT could result in losing two points from an application score overall, i.e. the equivalent to holding a 2.2 honours degree. The distribution of SJT scores from 2017 is shown in Fig. 4.1.

- Many students have objected to having to rank answers that are 'wrong'. Clearly this exercise does not hold very much practical relevance, although some might argue that this type of 'higher-order' thinking might help distinguish between candidates.
- The SJT asks what students *should* do, not what they *would* do (p. 12). It is debatable how relevant such a test can be in the absence of any way of measuring how someone *would* actually react, e.g. whether they are *actually* honest, virtuous, etc.

References and further reading

Halliwell-Ewen M, Lee C, Gopal D (2015). Deanery placement and the Situational Judgement Test. *Adv Med Educ Pract*, 6:631–2.

MacKenzie RK, Cleland JA, Ayansina D, Nicholson S (2016). Does the UKCAT predict performance on exit from medical school? A national cohort study. *BMJ Open*, 6:e011313.

MacKenzie RK, Dowell J, Ayansina D, Cleland JA (2017). Do personality traits assessed on medical school admission predict exit performance?

A UK-wide longitudinal cohort study. *Adv Health Sci Educ Theory Pract*, 22:365–85.

Najim M, Rabee R, Sherwani Y, *et al.* (2015). The situational judgement test: a student's worst nightmare. *Adv Med Educ Pract*, 6:577–8.

Petty-Saphon K, Walker K, Patterson F, Ashworth V, Edwards H (2017). Situational judgment tests reliably measure professional attributes important for clinical practice. *Adv Med Educ Pract*, 8:2–3.

Sharma N (2015). Medical students' perceptions of the situational judgement test: a mixed methods study. *Br J Hosp Med (Lond)*, 76:234–8.

Sharma N, Morgan M, Walsh K (2016). Faculty perception of the medical student situational judgement test – Summary of findings. *Med Teach*, 38:529.

Simon E, Walsh K, Paterson-Brown F, Cahill D (2015). Does a high ranking mean success in the Situational Judgement Test? *Clin Teach*, 12:42–5.

Walsh J, Harris B (2013). Situational Judgement Tests: more important than educational performance? *BMJ Careers*, 18th April 2013.

Chapter 5

How are SJT questions created?

The SJT questions were created following the professional attributes (p. 11) identified from the FY1 job analysis.

Question writing

Questions were written by volunteers at a series of dedicated workshops. The volunteers were not all doctors but should have been familiar with the FY1 role and have worked with junior doctors within the previous two years.

The ISFP Project Group employed 89 people to write SJT questions, of whom 69 (77.5%) were senior doctors, two (2.2%) were lay representatives, and the remainder were undeclared. In terms of background, 59 (66.3%) were from a range of acute specialties and 12 (13.5%) from community specialties.

Two-part review process

This team created a bank of 453 possible questions. These were scrutinized by a team of psychologists who accepted 360 questions as passing this initial stage.

A select few writers were asked to moderate all questions to ensure that scenarios were realistic and the terminology was in use across the UK. This group eliminated additional questions, leaving a total of 306.

Foundation doctor focus groups

A series of focus groups was then held with foundation doctors who scrutinized the test instructions and up to 20 questions each. They proposed a number of amendments and whittled down the total question bank to 275 items.

Concordance panel

Once a question bank was established, it was trialled using a panel of subject 'experts', i.e. people with similar qualifications to the question writers.

Questions survived this process if they achieved a satisfactory level of concordance, i.e. enough experts independently arrived at the same answer under test conditions. A total of 200 questions went forward to be used in the SJT pilots.

SJT pilots

The SJT model underwent two pilots. The second and larger of these took place in 13 UK medical schools, involving 639 final-year students. Students reported that the content seemed relevant to the Foundation Programme (85% agreed) and that the questions were fair (73.3%).

Why does this matter?

The reasons for understanding how questions are created are to appreciate the following:

- A lot of thought has gone into every question. There should be no ambiguities (unless intended) or 'tricks'.
- They are written (largely) by senior doctors who are presumably interested in medical training and development. This is the perspective informing both questions and answers.
- The question pool is relatively small as the number of possible scenarios is limited. This makes it easier to prepare for the SJT (p. 19) than might otherwise be imagined.

Chapter 6

How can you prepare?

The Improving Selection to the Foundation Programme (ISFP) project does not believe that it is possible to be 'coached' through the SJT. This is generally true. Knowing the 'right thing to do' in any given situation is a matter of internalized values and intuition.

However, no one seriously accepts that candidates are born with a fixed level of situational judgement. This is clearly something that develops over time and therefore can change.

In addition, the SJT does not set out to test *your* values but whether you *understand* the values and attitudes expected of an FY1 doctor. This is why you are instructed to answer questions as you 'should', not as you 'would'.

The principles on which foundation doctors should base their behaviour are learnt and internalized throughout medical school. However, knowledge of these principles can clearly be learnt in the same way as any other part of the medical school curriculum.

Is the SJT worth preparing for?

Most final-year medical students are satisfied with the FY1 posts to which they are allocated. For 2017 entry, 74% were appointed to their first-choice foundation school, and 94% to one of their top five preferences. Those who were not initially pleased often look back in retrospect and are satisfied with their allocations. Your score on the SJT is unlikely to make or break your career.

However, the same can be said of medical school finals. You will almost certainly pass finals—upwards of 95% of final-year students do so—and your ultimate career destination is unlikely to hinge on your cumulative examination score. But this is *not* a reason to go into finals unprepared.

The truth is that every point on the SJT, as in finals, could mean the difference between your chosen outcome and something different. A point lost on the SJT could result in your leaving your first-choice foundation school and moving across the country for work, or not having a high enough score to capture your chosen specialty as a Foundation Programme rotation.

Increasing competition for FY1 posts means that not everyone can be appointed. In some years, medical students have been placed on a reserve list, with no certainty of being offered a place on the Foundation Programme following qualification. Although all students on the reserve list have—so far—been placed eventually, you will want to avoid such uncertainty when preparing for your final exams. Although it only affects a small number in a pool of ~7000 applicants, it should be taken seriously.

Although you may be told otherwise, the SJT *is* a high-stakes examination. If other students choose not to maximize their score ('because you can't prepare for this type of test ... '), this is your opportunity to step ahead of the curve. If your colleagues are preparing, you need to redouble your efforts.

How can you prepare?

The values, attitudes, and behaviours expected of new doctors are helpfully recorded in a set of publicly available documents.

SJT question writers, whether explicitly or otherwise, will have internalized these principles over many years and used them to inform their answers. When doubt arose about the correct answer, these principles would have been definitive.

At some point in your preparation, you should read the following four documents:

- General Medical Council (www.gmc-uk.org):
  - *Good Medical Practice* (2013)
  - *Tomorrow's Doctors* (2009), particularly 'Outcomes 3—the Doctor as a Professional'.
- UK Foundation Programme (www.foundationprogramme.nhs.uk)
  - *Person Specification for Recruitment to the Foundation Programme*
  - *Foundation Programme Curriculum.*

As you read, you may feel that each statement is 'obvious'. This is because you began internalizing their contents years ago. Try to concentrate though, as their balance of priorities may be subtly different and shift your understanding, whether or not you realize this at the time.

If you have time, the GMC produces a vast amount of guidance, all of which could aid your approach to the SJT. The following documents, available electronically from the GMC website, might be useful:

- *0–18 Years: Guidance for All Doctors* (2007)
- *Confidentiality: Good Practice in Handling Patient Information* (2017)
- *Accountability in Multi-Disciplinary and Multi-Agency Mental Health Teams* (2005)
- *Confidentiality* (2009)
- *Consent: Patients and Doctors Making Decisions Together* (2008)
- *Good Practice in Prescribing Medicines* (2008)
- *Good Practice in Research and Consent to Research* (2010)
- *Leadership and Management for All Doctors* (2012)
- *Maintaining Boundaries* (2006)
- *Outcomes for Provisionally Registered Doctors With a Licence to Practice* (2015)
- *Personal Beliefs and Medical Practice* (2008)
- *Raising and Acting on Concerns About Patient Safety* (2012)
- *Reporting Convictions: Reporting Criminal and Regulatory Proceedings Within and Outside the UK* (2008)
- *Treatment and Care Towards the End of Life* (2010).

What about practice questions?

This is a book of practice questions. There are two ways that completing SJT-type questions will help you to maximize your score:

- Completing questions is a more active process than reading policy documents. Choosing the correct answer requires concentration. This will help you to internalize the values and attitudes described previously (p. 11). Seeing our explanations will make you think harder about the issues, particularly if you disagree with our answers!
- You will begin to intuitively spot phrases that indicate the appropriateness of each answer.

There are only 275 items in the official SJT question bank. This is because there are a limited number of realistic scenarios that can be imagined as happening to FY1 doctors. This book presents over 275 questions and there is likely to be considerable overlap. Complete all of these questions and you will have thought (reasonably) hard about every scenario that you will encounter in the SJT.

Tips for the SJT

1. Put yourself in the position of a new FY1 doctor when answering each question. But remember that they are asking what you *should* do, not what you *would* do.
2. You should be a paragon of virtue when answering all questions. Remember always that you are unfailingly honest, respectful, open, and fair to colleagues, patients, and relatives alike. It is difficult to imagine scenarios with answers that would require you to be otherwise.
3. If a question involves patient safety (e.g. critically unwell patient, drug error, etc.), your priority must *always* be making the patient safe.
4. The well-being of your patient is your first priority. Other considerations (e.g. relatives, targets, fear of being told off, going home on time) are always secondary.
5. 'Seeking senior advice' and 'gathering information' are difficult to criticize and tend to be safe options. Similarly, it is rarely incorrect to document events or complete a formal incident form.
6. Remember your limitations. As an FY1 doctor, you should not usually break bad news, consent patients for operations, administer cytotoxic or anaesthetic drugs, or manage critically ill patients without support. 'Call a senior' is the correct answer in these cases.
7. Understand basic concepts of medical law, e.g. when confidentiality can be breached, determining incapacity, consent in children, the doctrine of double effect, and detention under the Mental Health Act. You do not need to know specifics (e.g. sections of Acts), but a practical understanding will guide some answers.
8. As an FY1 doctor, your Clinical Supervisor is usually a consultant for whom you work during a particular rotation. They are an appropriate source of support for clinical development and problems within the team. Your Educational Supervisor is akin to a Personal Tutor, i.e. responsible for your overall welfare and development throughout the year. They can advise on pastoral issues, professional development, and difficulties with your Clinical Supervisor.
9. Try to complete all questions within the given time frame as random guesses may be identified by the scoring software and awarded zero (p. 10).

Chapter 8

How to use this book

Section 2 of this book is organized into five chapters, each representing a professional attribute to which SJT questions are mapped: commitment to professionalism (Chapter 9, p. 29), coping with pressure (Chapter 10, p. 71), effective communication (Chapter 11, p. 111), patient focus (Chapter 12, p. 149), and working effectively as part of a team (Chapter 13, p. 189). Each section contains 40 questions, split equally between multiple choice and ranking items. The book ends with Section 3, which contains abbreviated practice tests (Chapter 14, p. 231) that use a mix of different questions.

You will notice throughout the book that most questions cover multiple domains. This is true for those in the SJT as well. It is easy to imagine scenarios that test all five domains with very little effort; for example, a senior nurse pressures you to do something to the detriment of a patient. Do not become distracted by trying to guess which domain(s) are being tested.

Although the SJT requires knowledge (p. 11), the answers to questions cannot be learnt by rote. This is what the test creators mean when they say candidates cannot be 'coached' to score highly. The benefit in working through these examples is thinking about the issues they raise. For this reason, the 'wrong' answers are at least as valuable as those that are 'correct'.

When practising questions in other subjects (e.g. anatomy), most students read the question, choose an answer, and then check that they picked correctly. The best approach to this book is to read a scenario and then consciously think about which details make (C) a better choice than (D), or vice versa. Only when you have done this should you check our answer and explanation.

SJT questions go through a commendably thorough process of assessment and evaluation (p. 17). The answers are determined by a consensus panel of 'experts', most of whom are senior doctors.

Our own questions have been through an abbreviated review process using the contributors listed on p. xix–xx. This group of contributors broadly reflects the type of people used by the SJT team to validate their items, i.e. members include Clinical Supervisors, doctors with recent experience of the Foundation Programme, and others working closely with FY1 doctors (e.g. senior nurses). Despite our checks, you may disagree with some answers. Hopefully the accompanying explanation will convince you otherwise, but there is certainly room for disagreement. As long as you have carefully considered the issues raised by each question, it has fulfilled its purpose.

As you work through the questions, you will notice that certain themes arise again and again. This is because, although the facts of each scenario are infinite, only a small number of values and attitudes are expected of FY1 doctors. This explains why there are only 275 items in the SJT question bank (p. 17). Once questions feel repetitive, you have probably begun to identify the most appropriate answers intuitively. You might then be persuaded to try the practice test (p. 231).

A couple of health warnings

There are no 'right' and 'wrong' SJT answers. This is particularly frustrating for students who have spent years training to match factual recall (e.g. features of chronic heart failure) to factual situations (e.g. ankle oedema, breathlessness on exertion) with which they are presented. Unfortunately, this assessment tool has become another obstacle that must be surpassed to progress with your career. The SJT was not created by the editors of this book and neither would it have been their choice of tool with which to discriminate between candidates.

It is inevitable after such a test that candidates leave the exam room confident that they *should* have scored 100%. This is because each person naturally believes they could justify their answers if required. You will have the same feeling as you work through this book and the explanations may often be insufficient to persuade you that our chosen sequence was 'correct'. This will inevitably become a frustrating, uncomfortable, and unrewarding experience if taken personally.

You should not take the fact that your answers and ours do not match as any claim that your sequence is 'wrong'. It is quite feasible that you might disagree with our proposed sequence and be right every time. The editors do not claim any hidden knowledge or monopoly on moral truth and have only created these items as a vehicle to help students think through important professional issues.

It is particularly important that you do not become discouraged by small differences (e.g. whether option (C) should be in third or fourth place) as it is big discrepancies that are penalized most heavily by the SJT mark scheme (p. 10). If you cannot resolve a small difference, then accept that it does not matter and move on to another question.

A related health warning relates to the trap of 'memorizing' answers, as practice scenarios will never identically mirror those in the SJT. In medical school exams, you can sometimes latch on to keywords that announce the correct answer. For example, seeing 'Grey–Turner's sign' in a question stem might be sufficient by itself for your choice of 'haemorrhagic pancreatitis' as the cause of abdominal pain in a surgery multiple choice exam. However, this technique does not translate well to the SJT. You cannot summarize a question stem as 'drunk consultant' and safely assume the answer is 'to contact the Clinical Director', just because this is recommended in a similar practice question. The little details and precise wording of answers *matter* for SJT-type questions, so don't get caught out.

Section 2

Questions

Chapter 9

Commitment
to professionalism

Introduction

The Royal College of Physicians (RCP) has defined professionalism as a 'set of values, behaviours, and relationships that underpins the trust the public has in doctors'. Dame Janet Smith has described professionalism as 'a basket of qualities that enables us to trust our advisors'. The RCP has imagined some of the qualities that might be included within Dame Janet's basket as 'integrity, compassion, altruism, continuous improvement, excellence, and working in partnership'. The General Medical Council (GMC) has taken this further in the 'Professionalism in action' section of *Good Medical Practice* (2013). According to the GMC, good doctors 'make the care of their patients their first concern: they are competent, keep their knowledge and skills up to date, establish and maintain good relationships with patients and colleagues, are honest and trustworthy, and act with integrity and within the law. They also work in partnership with patients and respect their rights to privacy and dignity. They treat each patient as an individual. They do their best to make sure all patients receive good care and treatment that will support them to live as well as possible, whatever their illness or disability'.

The Medical Protection Society (MPS) has, however, been clear that 'professionalism' is not the same as 'perfectionism'. Although professionalism encompasses the ambition to provide high-quality care, mistakes are an inevitable part of working as a doctor. For the MPS, 'true professionalism comes into play when mistakes are made ... knowing what to do when things go wrong and how to react appropriately can make all the difference in ensuring high standards of patient care are maintained and a speedy resolution is reached'.

Situational judgement questions within this section will test your probity by exploring responses to scenarios that might require you to challenge unacceptable behaviour, maintain confidentiality, and, as always, prioritize patient safety. You need to demonstrate a commitment to achieving your various clinical responsibilities, as well as a desire for continued learning and a commitment to helping the development of others. These scenarios test your honesty towards patients and colleagues, and a willingness to admit mistakes.

Other commonly recurring themes in this section will be social media and confidentiality. The former is ubiquitous and a relatively frequent means by which junior doctors (amongst other professionals) can get into trouble. A number of bodies—including the GMC and the British Medical Association (BMA)—have issued social media guidance that is specific to doctors. You might find some of the advice (e.g. always identifying yourself by name if presenting yourself as a doctor on social media) to be surprisingly restrictive.

A doctor acting professionally will:

- always honour their clinical commitments
- avoid rude or disrespectful behaviour
- challenge unsatisfactory clinical standards in a way that is firm but proportionate
- avoid gossip and unwarranted criticism or patients or colleagues
- ensure they have appropriate training or expertise before undertaking a procedure
- respond positively to feedback and learn from mistakes
- avoid behaviour that undermines the standing of the profession, even if that behaviour was arguably acceptable in some other sense
- strive to do the *right* thing, even when that is difficult or may lead to conflict.

A few tips that are specific to questions testing this domain:

- These questions will set up circumstances designed to distract you from acting professionally. Do not be fooled.
- Always be willing to challenge unprofessional behaviour exhibited by colleagues, but do so in an appropriate manner.
- Be open about your mistakes to both colleagues and patients. Never be tempted to 'cover up' errors, whether they are your own or a colleague's.

Importantly, professionalism is the thread that runs through all five domains that are tested by the SJT. This opening chapter is therefore a good time to start reading and internalizing some of the work that has already been published on professionalism. We recommend reading through the following documents, as well as using practice SJT questions, to get you thinking about professional attitudes and behaviours. If the URLs provided under 'References and further reading' are 'broken', then all the documents should be freely accessible by searching for their titles using a mainstream search engine.

References and further reading

British Medical Association (2017). *Social Media, Ethics and Professionalism*. https://www.bma.org.uk/advice/employment/ethics/social-media-guidance-for-doctors

General Medical Council (2013). *Doctors' Use of Social Media*. http://www.gmc-uk.org/Doctors__use_of_social_media.pdf_51448306.pdf

General Medical Council (2013). *Good Medical Practice*. http://www.gmc-uk.org/guidance/good_medical_practice/professionalism_in_action.asp

Medical Protection Society (2015). *Professionalism: A Medical Protection Guide*. http://www.medicalprotection.org/docs/default-source/pdfs/Booklet-PDFs/professionalism-a-medical-protection-guide.pdf

Royal College of Physicians (2005). *Doctors in Society: Medical Professionalism in a Changing World*. https://shop.rcplondon.ac.uk/products/doctors-in-society-medical-professionalism-in-a-changing-world

QUESTIONS

1. A junior colleague on your team always takes his copy of the patient list home as there is no confidential waste bin on the ward. He says this also helps him prepare for the following day as he can memorize details in time for the consultant ward round.

Rank in order the following actions in response to this situation (1 = Most appropriate; 5 = Least appropriate)

A Tell him this is unfair as he is 'getting ahead' and making you look disorganized by knowing patient details before the ward round.

B Ask Matron or a Senior Sister about obtaining a confidential waste bin.

C Let your colleague know that he should not be taking a patient list home each day.

D Speak to the consultant about your colleague's behaviour.

E Take your own list home so that you can be as familiar with the patients as your colleague.

2. A patient on your ward is HIV-positive. He is from a minority community which he feels might react negatively if they knew of his diagnosis. As a result, he is very anxious that no one (including his close family) should be told.

Rank in order the following actions in response to this situation (1 = Most appropriate; 5 = Least appropriate)

A Eliminate all mention of HIV from his notes.

B Amend your patient list so this detail is missing or obscured (e.g. 'retroviral illness').

C Ensure the safety of other doctors and phlebotomists by writing 'HIV+' on blood requests.

D Tell the patient that he should talk to his family as you cannot guarantee complete confidentiality.

E Continue as you would for any other patient under your care.

3. You are sitting in the pub opposite your hospital after work. A group of doctors and nurses from another department is talking loudly and joking about patients on their ward. These patients could easily be identified from the conversations you are overhearing.

Rank in order the following actions in response to this situation (1 = Most appropriate; 5 = Least appropriate)

A Speak to the person who is speaking loudest so he is aware that his behaviour is inappropriate.

B Call hospital security and ask them to intervene.

C Challenge the whole group so that they are aware that their behaviour is inappropriate.

D Contact a manager in their department the following day to alert them to this breach.

E Ignore the situation, as they should know better and you do not want to cause a scene.

4. As you arrive on the ward one morning, you hear a nurse in a side room shouting at a patient. The tone and language used are unpleasant. You know that the patient is elderly and has severe dementia.

Rank in order the following actions in response to this situation (1 = Most appropriate; 5 = Least appropriate)

A Knock on the door and ask to speak with the nurse.

B Discuss the issue with a senior nurse (e.g. Matron) in the first instance as soon as they arrive.

C Make preliminary enquiries from other staff working that night to ask if they have noticed inappropriate behaviour.

D Use body language to show your disapproval, but do nothing formally as patient safety is not at risk.

E Contact the Care Quality Commission anonymously to avoid raising the issue with employees of your Trust.

5. You begin induction at your new Trust and are asked to sign a number of agreements. One of these is an agreement never to raise concerns with bodies outside of your employing organization. This is a condition of taking up your post.

Rank in order the following actions in response to this situation (1 = Most appropriate; 5 = Least appropriate)

A Sign the form and begin work as instructed.

B Throw the form away and hope that no one notices that it was not returned.

C Explain that you cannot sign as this prohibits you raising concerns appropriately about patient welfare.

D Sign the form, but resolve to raise concerns about patient safety in whatever way is necessary to ensure their resolution.

E Contact your medical defence organization or the GMC for advice if in doubt.

6. You are on call and asked to prescribe amoxicillin for a patient complaining of pain on urination. The nurse has tested his urine which shows leucocytes and nitrites characteristic of a urinary tract infection. Amoxicillin is the suggested treatment according to local protocol.

Rank in order the following actions in response to this situation (1 = Most appropriate; 5 = Least appropriate)

A Thank the nurse for being proactive and prescribe amoxicillin.

B Prescribe trimethoprim as this is the antibiotic of choice according to your recollections from medical school.

C Review the patient yourself and then prescribe if necessary.

D Reprimand the nurse for testing the urine without instruction.

E Explain that you will only prescribe antibiotics if the patient becomes confused or haemodynamically compromised.

7. You feel understaffed and undersupported when on call. Together with an FY2 doctor, you are responsible for all new medical admissions and the welfare of around 300 ward patients. Attempts to raise your concern with managers, your Educational Supervisor, and the Clinical Director have been unsuccessful.

Rank in order the following actions in response to this situation (1 = Most appropriate; 5 = Least appropriate)

A Contact the Medical Director and, if necessary, the Trust Chairman.

B Document each stage of your complaint carefully.

C Contact a documentary programme and offer to carry a hidden camera to capture specific problems.

D Write an article for your local newspaper raising concerns about the care of Mrs Baggins in side room 4.

E Carry on and do your best whenever you are on call.

8. Your consultant knows that you are interested in his specialty and suggests that you attend a one-day course in another city the following week. You recognize that this would be a good opportunity for professional development. Unfortunately you have no remaining annual leave days and are not entitled to study leave. The rota administrator says that you cannot have time off to attend.

Rank in order the following actions in response to this situation (1 = Most appropriate; 5 = Least appropriate)

A Ask your Senior House Officer (SHO) if she will look after the ward in your absence and go if she agrees.

B Speak to your Educational Supervisor and, with their support, ask the service manager for special permission.

C Accept that you cannot attend the course.

D Add up the number of days that you worked late the week before and attend the course as you are owed enough hours in lieu.

E Attend the course as you already have your consultant's permission.

9. An elderly patient's daughter tells you that she is concerned about the ward care of her mother. She is thinking about writing a formal complaint and asks you if she is over-reacting and how best to complain.

Rank in order the following actions in response to this situation (1 = Most appropriate; 5 = Least appropriate)

A Tell her that you will look into things but that a formal complaint will not help.

B Suggest that she drops into the Patient Advice and Liaison Service (PALS) to see what they can offer.

C Explore her concerns and try to clear up any misunderstandings.

D Let your consultant and/or the Ward Sister know that the daughter is dissatisfied and that a formal complaint might follow.

E Tell the daughter that the ward nurses are particularly bad and that she should complain.

10. You are reviewing the drug chart of Tim, a young male patient with a previous anaphylactic reaction to penicillin. Your registrar has prescribed Tazocin® which you know contains a penicillin antibiotic. The patient has not yet received his first dose.

Rank in order the following actions in response to this situation (1 = Most appropriate; 5 = Least appropriate)

A Strike out the prescription and let the nurse know that it should not be administered.

B Complete a clinical incident form.

C Speak with the registrar to alert him/her to this error.

D Ensure that the allergy is recorded clearly on the drug chart and in the patient's notes.

E Amend the prescription, but do not cause a fuss as no harm was done.

11. You are concerned that patients on your ward are rarely seen by a senior doctor. They are reviewed weekly by a registrar but almost never by consultants, who seem to be working at a private hospital most of the time. You are uncertain whether to raise the issue or how you would do this as both your Clinical and Educational Supervisors are consultants within this department. You are deciding whom to contact for advice.

Choose the THREE most appropriate actions to take in this situation

A The consultant who seems most absent from the department and is known to have the biggest private practice.

B Your partner.

C Your medical defence organization.

D A friend from school whose judgement you trust and is now a solicitor.

E An employer liaison officer at the General Medical Council.

F A consultant in another department who is known for his fierce opposition to private practice.

G An SHO who spends his weekends at the private hospital assisting in theatre.

H A senior non-clinical colleague (e.g. a manager).

12. A medical student approaches you for advice. He is very concerned that your consultant has asked students to perform rectal examinations on patients under general anaesthesia without consent. You doubt that this is possible and suspect consent must have been obtained beforehand.

Choose the THREE most appropriate actions to take in this situation

A Warn the student not to say anything as he will upset the consultant and/or make him angry.

B Explain that the consultant is very professional and that consent might have been obtained beforehand.

C Explain that consent was probably obtained beforehand and that the student should do as instructed in theatre.

D Advise the student to ask the consultant if there is doubt about the consent process.

E Warn the student not to say anything as he needs the consultant's support to pass the rotation.

F Tell the student that specific consent for him is not required for some procedures (e.g. rectal cancer resection).

G Advise the student to mention this on the anonymous feedback after the rotation ends.

H Suggest that the student speaks to an appropriate person at his medical school if in doubt.

13. You are the surgical FY1 doctor and hear that an unconscious patient in the A&E resuscitation area has a ruptured abdominal aortic aneurysm (AAA). Your SHO tells you to feel the patient's abdomen as this is a rare opportunity to feel the expansile mass about which you read in textbooks. You have never felt a ruptured AAA before.

Choose the THREE most appropriate actions to take in this situation

A Decline to examine the patient as you do not have consent.

B Make a note to read about AAAs as this is not something you have encountered properly before.

C Find your medical students so that they can examine the patient as well.

D Examine the patient as this is a valuable learning opportunity.

E Introduce yourself to the most senior doctor present and ask if you can examine the patient.

F Tell your SHO that you are busy on the ward and will go later if you have time.

G Call the patient's next of kin at home to ask if you can examine her father. .

H Tell your SHO that you will only examine the patient if he completes a work-based assessment for your e-portfolio.

14. You are a medical FY1 doctor seeing a new patient in A&E. This could be an opportunity to ask your senior to complete a work-based assessment for your e-portfolio. The assessment requires a senior doctor to observe you examining a patient and then complete an electronic form. You ask the medical registrar who says she is too busy to help. Your SHO overhears and offers to complete the assessment without seeing you examine the patient.

Choose the THREE most appropriate actions to take in this situation

A Thank the registrar and ask if you could present the case to her later for your own experience.

B Tell the registrar that you need senior feedback if you are to develop as a doctor.

C Thank the SHO and forward him an electronic form to complete.

D Ask the SHO if he will complete two work-based assessments at the same time.

E Ask the SHO to watch you examine the patient and then complete an assessment.

F Examine the patient as formally as possible, even though you are not being assessed.

G Examine the patient a few hours later when someone might be available to assess you.

H Tell your Educational Supervisor how difficult it is to get senior colleagues to complete formal assessments.

15. You are an FY1 doctor required to attend mandatory teaching on Tuesday afternoon. This is also the time that your consultant holds his only ward round of the week. Your registrar is unimpressed that you want to 'slip off' when you are needed to update the consultant on each patient's progress. He suggests that you sign the attendance register, then return to the ward round.

Choose the THREE most appropriate actions to take in this situation

A Explain that teaching is mandatory and you are required to attend.

B Sign the attendance register so that your progression through FY1 is not obstructed, and then attend the ward round.

C Agree that your presence on the ward round is necessary and that you will miss teaching.

D Speak with your consultant and explain that your commitments are conflicting.

E Offer to update your registrar about each patient so that he can facilitate the ward round in your place.

F Explain that teaching is mandatory and then go to the doctors' mess for a long break.

G Attend the ward round, but read up on the teaching you missed afterwards.

H Send a text message asking an FY1 colleague to sign you in to teaching.

16. Your consultant has two third-year medical students and asks you to teach them for a day. You are a new FY1 doctor who is not yet confident with the role and feel that you are too busy to look after students.

Choose the THREE most appropriate actions to take in this situation

A Tell your consultant that you are far too busy to look after students.

B Wait until your consultant has left, and then sign the students' attendance forms and send them away.

C Wait until your consultant has left and then tell the students that you are too busy.

D Give your bleep to a colleague and deliver a 60-minute tutorial on a topic of your choice.

E Explore the students' career aspirations and ask what jobs they are applying for.

F Give the students clear tasks that match their learning objectives and help you if possible.

G Ask the students to spend the morning completing discharge summaries which you will check and sign afterwards.

H Ask the students questions about topics with which you are particularly comfortable.

17. You are coming to the end of FY1 and are being shadowed by the final-year medical student intended to replace you. You are very concerned about his attitude towards other healthcare professionals and have received negative feedback from the nursing staff. After five weeks, he asks you to complete a feedback form for his medical school.

Choose the THREE most appropriate actions to take in this situation

A Tell the student throughout the placement that he should adjust his attitude.

B Wait until the end of the placement and then meet somewhere privately to discuss your concerns.

C Tell the student about your concerns, but mark all performance domains as 'satisfactory'.

D Let your Clinical Supervisor know that the incoming FY1 doctor has a bad attitude.

E Indicate your concerns on the feedback form with specific examples.

F Give the student an opportunity to discuss your feedback.

G Write to the medical school dean suggesting that formal action be considered.

H Wish the nursing staff 'good luck' working with the incoming FY1 doctor.

18. Your Trust has introduced mandatory online prescribing training for specific drugs (e.g. insulin, warfarin, and antibiotics).

You are confident working with these drugs and will probably have to complete the training in your own time as your ward commitments are excessive.

Choose the THREE most appropriate actions to take in this situation

A Decline to complete the online modules because there is no time during your working day.

B Complete the online modules quickly, but pick random answers so that you don't have to read the text.

C Ask your Clinical Supervisor or an appropriate manager for protected time in which to complete the modules.

D Complete the modules in your own time without complaint.

E Refuse to complete the modules, but satisfy yourself that you can prescribe safely.

F Provide feedback after completing the modules as to whether or not you found them helpful.

G Ask your partner, who is a doctor, to complete the modules for you at home while you are on call.

H Contact the British Medical Association to ask whether you can be forced to complete the modules.

19. A group of five medical students is attached to your firm. You have been spending a lot of time with one of the students and feel that a mutual attraction is developing.

Choose the THREE most appropriate actions to take in this situation

A Try to avoid the student for the rest of the rotation.

B Meet with the student socially so that any romance can develop away from the workplace.

C Try to ensure that your attention is equally distributed between all students on the firm.

D Avoid any romance developing while the student is attached to your firm.

E Tell the student that you are attracted to them but that you should remain professional.

F Ask one of the others whether this particular student is attracted to you.

G Try to avoid unprofessional feelings developing in future.

H Continue with any developing relationship, as you are not directly responsible for supervising medical students.

20. You have been looking after Sid, a 90-year-old with end-stage heart failure, for a number of months. His condition is worsening. You visit one day and he hands you an envelope containing £500. Although you protest, he insists, saying that it is a 'thank you' and that he 'doesn't need it any more'.

Choose the THREE most appropriate actions to take in this situation

A Tell Sid that the gift is too much and that you will only accept £50.

B Thank Sid for the gift, but explain that you are unable to accept.

C Accept the gift and then ask an appropriate person within the Trust whether this is allowed.

D Ask Sid to sign a statement so you are not accused of theft later on.

E Accept the gift, but give it to Sid's daughter, who is his next of kin, at her next visit.

F Ask him to think carefully about his decision.

G Suggest that he donates the money to your favourite charity instead.

H Ask an appropriate person in the Trust for advice.

21. As the obstetrics and gynaecology FY1 doctor, you are called to see a 30-year-old woman who is four hours postpartum and is actively bleeding. The patient is a Jehovah's Witness and she tells you she will not accept any blood products. Despite your attempts at fluid resuscitation, the patient continues to bleed. She remains hypotensive, with an Hb of 5.5, although still alert and orientated.

Choose the THREE most appropriate actions to take in this situation

A Transfuse her immediately with red blood cells.

B The woman's decision can be overruled when a child's life is at risk.

C Commence a frank discussion with the patient, highlighting the risks and benefits of the blood transfusion, including the possibility of death if she refuses.

D Continue to give intravenous fluids if the patient consents, but do not transfuse any blood products.

E Wait until the patient becomes unconscious before attempting to transfuse blood products.

F Seek the advice of the consultant haematologist as soon as possible.

G Call the Hospital Liaison Committee for Jehovah's Witnesses.

H Speak to your consultant to initiate the process of overruling the patient's decision with a court order.

22. You are examining a ten-month-old infant in A&E who has been brought in by his parents after an episode of bloody diarrhoea. On examination, you find that he has significant scarring secondary to his circumcision. The parents say that the circumcision was performed by an experienced religious leader in accordance with their beliefs.

Rank in order the following actions in response to this situation (1 = Most appropriate; 5 = Least appropriate)

A The scarring does not require treatment on this admission, as it has nothing to do with the presenting complaint.

B Document the findings and discuss the management options with your consultant.

C The examination finding constitutes evidence of genital mutilation, and Child Protection Services should be informed immediately.

D Refer the patient to a paediatric surgeon for further assessment.

E Refer the parents to parenting classes for failing to act in accordance with their child's best interests.

23. You receive your first pay cheque as a qualified doctor at the end of a very busy month's work on an understaffed medical ward. You are pleasantly surprised to find that you have received substantial payment for locum shifts, despite having never been asked to work outside your contracted hours. You calculate that the additional hours you have had to work on the medical ward approximate to the additional payment you have received in error.

Rank in order the following actions in response to this situation (1 = Most appropriate; 5 = Least appropriate)

A Overall, you are receiving the correct amount of payment and are not under any obligation to correct an error made by payroll.

B Write a cheque amounting to 95% of the total additional income that you have been paid for a charity of your choice, retaining a small amount as compensation for your efforts.

C Keep a work diary of the number of hours that you are working.

D Involve your Educational Supervisor, as you should not be working outside your contracted hours.

E Alert payroll to the error so that any additional payment can be docked from your salary.

24. You are preparing your specialty training application for general surgery. You had few opportunities to gain experience in theatre as a foundation doctor. However, you have spoken to many people about surgical careers and watched video recordings of operations. You have booked a Basic Surgical Skills course and read the manual, but have yet to attend it. You are considering what statements you can legitimately make on your application.

Choose the THREE most appropriate actions to take in this situation

A I have enjoyed participating in various operations during my time as a foundation doctor.

B I have enjoyed developing my surgical knowledge through experience as a foundation doctor.

C While I have made every effort to learn about a career in surgery, my Foundation Programme rotations have not allowed time to attend theatre.

D I have managed to gain indirect experience of theatre through watching videos of operations in my spare time.

E I have developed an enthusiasm for the working environment of the operating room through extensive surgical experience.

F I look forward to developing my surgical experience during this surgical specialty training programme.

G I am fully proficient in the Basic Surgical Skills course curriculum.

H My inexperience in the operating room is compensated by a superior command of general medicine.

25. You are completing an orthopaedics audit during one of your FY1 rotations. The consultant surgeon has asked you to review the complication rates for total knee replacements performed at this hospital and compare them with the average across the Trust. Your analysis shows slightly worse post-operative outcomes at this hospital, and the average appears to be significantly skewed by the high complication rates of your consultant.

Rank in order the following actions in response to this situation (1 = Most appropriate; 5 = Least appropriate)

A Report the consultant surgeon to the Care Quality Commission, as this is an issue of patient safety.

B Ask all the orthopaedic consultants for advice about the data at the following week's departmental meeting.

C Speak with your consultant orthopaedic surgeon privately about the findings.

D Omit your consultant's data, and submit a report without further discussion.

E Obtain further data on preoperative parameters for the cases.

26. After leaving your evening shift as the on-call medical FY1 doctor, you walk through the town and come across a group of medical students who have been attached to your ward. They are behaving quite out of character, obviously under the influence of alcohol, and are shouting profanities at passers-by. The students are eventually confronted by a passing police officer before being asked to move on.

Choose the THREE most appropriate actions to take in this situation

A No further action is necessary, as medical students are not regulated by the same code of practice as doctors.

B Chase the students down the street and demand that they answer for their actions.

C Inform your Educational Supervisor about what has occurred in the morning.

D Email details of what you observed to the medical school dean.

E Approach the police officer and enquire as to whether further action is needed.

F Confront the medical students about their behaviour the following day.

G Reserve your comments until the end of their medical placement when you are asked to give formal written feedback.

H Withhold any details of the incident from other junior colleagues.

27. During a two-week vacation in Singapore, you became embroiled in an altercation at a bar and were subsequently given a caution by police. You return to work feeling rather upset and ashamed, but determined to put the whole incident behind you.

Rank in order the following actions in response to this situation (1 = Most appropriate; 5 = Least appropriate)

A Try to put the issue behind you.

B Wait until you have settled into your new rotation before raising the issue.

C Inform your Medical Defence Union and seek legal advice.

D Contact the GMC immediately to report the caution.

E Ask your consultant for advice as to how you should proceed.

28. You arrive at work before the consultant ward round and attempt to print the patient list. You are hindered by slow equipment and a broken printer. The ward round is unable to begin until you have a current patient list and your consultant is frustrated as he needs to begin an all-day endoscopy list.

Rank in order the following actions in response to this situation (1 = Most appropriate; 5 = Least appropriate)

A Express your frustration with the IT equipment and demand that the consultant requests replacements.

B Send the patient list to your personal email address and print it on the neighbouring ward.

C Ask a medical student to print the list while you begin the ward round.

D Ask the nurses on each of the wards whether there are any new patients who are under the care of your consultant.

E Advise the team to reconvene in 15 minutes while you contact the IT helpdesk and attempt to print the list.

29. You observe an FY1 colleague shouting at a staff nurse in front of a patient. Afterwards, the nurse approaches you to discuss the FY1 doctor's behaviour. He explains that the FY1 has had several 'angry outbursts' since joining the ward two months ago and he is unsure how to deal with them.

Rank in order the following actions in response to this situation (1 = Most appropriate; 5 = Least appropriate)

A Advise the nurse to talk to his line manager as it is not your responsibility to get involved in nursing-related matters.

B Bleep the FY1 and ask him to return to the ward and apologize to the nurse and patient.

C Apologize on behalf of the FY1, and ask the nurse not to pursue the matter any further at this time as you will speak to the other doctor.

D Inform the FY1 colleague's Clinical Supervisor about the episode and what the staff nurse has told you.

E Send an email to your FY1 colleague detailing what the staff nurse has told you, to provide a written record of your conversation.

30. During the return flight from your holiday abroad, an announcement is made requesting medical assistance for one of the passengers. You graduated from medical school three weeks ago and have yet to start your first job as an FY1 doctor; you feel particularly apprehensive about attending to a possible in-flight emergency on your own.

Rank in order the following actions in response to this situation (1 = Most appropriate; 5 = Least appropriate)

A Do nothing since you are not legally bound to provide medical assistance as you have not yet signed a contract with your employer.

B Inform the cabin crew that you are a recently qualified doctor, and begin your medical assessment immediately.

C Approach the unwell passenger and determine if you will be able to offer any help before informing the cabin crew of your presence.

D Wait for ten minutes to see if anyone else on board can assist before volunteering to assess the passenger.

E Review the passenger, but ask the cabin crew to make an announcement for more senior medical assistance as you are only recently qualified and very inexperienced.

31. A group of medical students ask if you can help them prepare for their forthcoming end-of-module examination on the respiratory system. You agree to teach them at the end of the week, provided that they stay and assist you with some ward jobs, which they agree to do. You are reminded about your teaching commitment the day before the students' examination, but unfortunately you have forgotten to prepare a relevant lesson plan.

Rank in order the following actions in response to this situation (1 = Most appropriate; 5 = Least appropriate)

A Inform the students that they should have reminded you earlier in the week, and now you are unable to teach them.

B Defer the teaching until they want to prepare for their next end-of-module examination.

C Attempt to teach the students, even if your knowledge is insufficient, but finish the teaching early if it does not prove helpful.

D Teach the students about haematology, with which you are more comfortable.

E Adopt a style of teaching that only utilizes questioning the students, and reflect every question asked back towards the group.

32. You are asked by your consultant in paediatric surgery to clerk an infant who has been admitted to A&E with bilious vomiting. This is the first week of your first FY1 rotation and you have had limited experience in paediatrics beyond your five-week rotation in medical school two years ago. You are unsure whether you should clerk the patient, if you should inform the parents of your inexperience, and who would be responsible if you were to assess the infant.

Choose the THREE most appropriate actions to take in this situation

A Attempt a rudimentary clerking before calling the consultant to review the patient.

B Refuse to clerk the patient as you do not have sufficient experience.

C Conduct a thorough assessment of the patient once you are sure that he is stable.

D Act with the knowledge that the consultant is ultimately responsible for your assessment, as his trainee.

E Act with the knowledge that you are responsible for your assessment of the patient.

F Introduce yourself as a doctor, but do not state your seniority for fear of further worrying the infant's parents.

G State your position as a junior doctor.

H Admit that this is your first week as a junior doctor but that you will not be responsible for any treatment decisions yourself.

33. The final-year medical student attached to your ward asks you if you could write a reference in support of his application for a university-level history course which starts three months before his final-year examinations. You are concerned as, despite his enthusiasm, the student has a poor clinical knowledge base. You are not convinced by his assurances that he will be able to balance this new commitment with his medical course.

Rank in order the following actions in response to this situation (1 = Most appropriate; 5 = Least appropriate)

A Write a reference indicating that his knowledge base is poor but that he might do much better in another academic subject.

B Write a supportive reference, as his clinical knowledge base is not relevant to his performance on a history course.

C Suggest that he asks your consultant to write a reference to provide a more seasoned perspective on his ability.

D Tell the student that your position might not qualify you to comment on his suitability for the course.

E Set the student a mock clinical examination, and offer to write his reference based on his performance.

34. A male FY1 colleague in paediatrics is clerking a frightened 15-year-old girl who has been brought into A&E by her older sister who says that she has been the victim of a violent attack. After establishing a good rapport with the patient, the FY1 arranges for a physical examination. However, the girl remains adamant that no one else be present. In the absence of your registrar, your fellow FY1 asks for your advice.

Rank in order the following actions in response to this situation (1 = Most appropriate; 5 = Least appropriate)

A Advise him not to examine the patient and instead wait for the registrar.

B Suggest that he performs a physical examination by inspection alone, with a chaperone present if the girl agrees.

C He should agree to forego the chaperone and complete a thorough physical and internal examination to rule out any genital injury.

D Tell him to insist on the presence of a female nurse as a chaperone, and to avoid examining the patient if she insists on no one else being present.

E Ask the older sister to sign in the medical notes agreeing to act as the chaperone.

35. Your hospital is at the centre of a news story regarding a leaked audit which shows a recent rise in mortality following heart valve replacements. As an FY1 doctor on the cardiothoracic ward, you feel strongly about the negative portrayal of your senior surgical colleagues' abilities, believing the results to be due to the use of a new prosthesis. A news reporter approaches you as you are leaving the ward and asks if you would like to comment.

Rank in order the following actions in response to this situation (1 = Most appropriate; 5 = Least appropriate)

A Share with the reporter your honest opinions of the competence of your senior colleagues and the possibility of a fault with the new prosthetic valves.

B Ask for the contact details of the reporter and agree to an interview once you have obtained permission from your local Trust.

C Politely decline to comment.

D Discuss in general terms the difficulty that surgical innovators face when introducing novel technologies, without going into specific details about your department.

E Explain your frustration with the ignorance demonstrated by the media and the general public in relation to health matters.

36. You have volunteered to be the deanery's FY1 representative. A recent survey has shown that the greatest frustration of 90% of FY1 doctors is the limited teaching given during a typical week. However, a senior member of the deanery committee has described his frustration at your 'difficult predecessor' who was constantly 'trying to change things', and you are unsure how receptive the committee will be to your suggestions.

Rank in order the following actions in response to this situation (1 = Most appropriate; 5 = Least appropriate)

A Based on the recent survey findings, request approval for a full review into the teaching provided for FY1 doctors by each hospital's postgraduate medical education office.

B Conduct another questionnaire asking more specific questions about the teaching to the FY1 doctors themselves.

C Avoid the topic during your initial committee meetings, as you are unlikely to gain the favour of your seniors.

D Predict the response of all of the FY1 doctors to questions on the failures of teaching based on your own experiences, and take this evidence to the committee as justification for a detailed review by each hospital's education office.

E Resign as the deanery's FY1 representative.

37. You are left a gift of substantial value from the family of a wealthy patient whom you have recently cared for on the ward. You are frequently praised for the time and effort that you spend with patients, but this is the first time that you have personally received a gift.

Rank in order the following actions in response to this situation (1 = Most appropriate; 5 = Least appropriate)

A Inform the GMC of the gift.

B Inform the Ward Sister in charge of the gift.

C Seek the advice of your medico-legal defence organization.

D Accept the gift, but share its monetary value with the rest of your medical team.

E Attempt to obtain the family's details and return the gift.

38. An FY1 doctor who works with you on the surgical ward is asked to complete a death certificate and cremation form for a patient he has been treating. However, he has a conscientious objection to cremation, based on religious beliefs, and would prefer you to complete the form, even though you have never met the patient.

Rank in order the following actions in response to this situation (1 = Most appropriate; 5 = Least appropriate)

A Agree to complete the cremation form, as your colleague has provided a valid reason for refusing.

B Advise your colleague to claim that he has not been adequately trained to complete cremation forms.

C Inform your colleague that he has a duty to put aside any personal beliefs and complete the cremation form.

D Suggest he takes a few days of annual leave which will give the bereavement office time to find someone else to complete the form.

E Refuse to sign the cremation form on the grounds that you are not familiar with the patient.

39. You are a foundation doctor with an interest in orthopaedic surgery. In an effort to improve your specialty training application, you would like to complete an Advanced Trauma Life Support (ATLS) course. Unfortunately, your Trust gives priority to doctors working in A&E. One of the A&E doctors has been given a place on this basis but offers it to you in exchange for covering one of his night shifts.

Rank in order the following actions in response to this situation (1 = Most appropriate; 5 = Least appropriate)

A Accept the offer as it appears to be a mutually beneficial agreement.

B Tell the other foundation doctor that you will gratefully accept his offer but you are not willing to complete the weekend shift.

C Refuse the offer.

D Ask the advice of the ATLS coordinator at your hospital.

E Accept his offer and attend the course, but do not turn up for the weekend shift.

40. As the FY1 doctor in cardiology, you are responsible for looking after your consultant's NHS patients. One of the patients who had been under your care for the last 48 hours is transferred to the private ward on the other side of the hospital. At the request of your consultant, the nurses on the private ward have bleeped you on several occasions to complete various clinical procedures. You feel challenged by the additional workload and are uncertain whether you will complete your routine tasks.

Rank in order the following actions in response to this situation (1 = Most appropriate; 5 = Least appropriate)

A Ask the consultant for additional reimbursement in return for providing more of your time for assisting with his private patients.

B Explain the situation to one of the other cardiology consultants.

C Speak to the patient and ask whether he would mind returning to the NHS ward.

D Arrange a meeting with the cardiology consultant, via his secretary, to discuss the additional workload.

E Do not respond to any bleeps from the private ward; if it is genuinely a consultant's request, he will contact you.

41. An audit reveals a consistent deterioration in clinical outcomes for stroke patients managed by the new consultant. He suggests that you probably made an error in your data collection and the results should be ignored.

Choose the THREE most appropriate actions to take in this situation

A Carefully re-check your data and any analyses.

B Consider the consultant's suggestion and avoid drawing any conclusions.

C Present the data at the departmental meeting.

D Challenge the consultant regarding his clinical outcomes.

E Survey the other consultants in the department privately about their interpretations of the data.

F Involve someone with more research experience to check for mistakes.

G Ask the next FY1 joining the team to repeat the audit in 4 months' time.

H Speak to another consultant, such as your Clinical Supervisor or the Clinical Director.

42. Your SHO asks you to prescribe some antibiotics for their partner.

Rank in order the following actions in response to this situation (1 = Most appropriate; 5 = Least appropriate)

A Politely decline.

B Suggest the partner comes in for you to examine them.

C Ask your colleague to speak with the registrar.

D Sign the prescription with false details so it can't be processed.

E Sign the prescription.

43. You have completed a research project looking at surgical outcomes in your department and are preparing an abstract for submission to a conference. A new registrar who has only just joined your department insists that she should be named as an author.

Choose the THREE most appropriate actions to take in this situation

A Inform the ethics department in the hospital.

B Contact the registrar's Educational Supervisor.

C Discuss the requirements for authorship and assess whether the registrar fulfils any of these.

D Refuse.

E Offer authorship for this work with the promise that she will assist in any future project or publication.

F Invite the registrar to make comments and changes to the abstract in exchange for her authorship.

G Confront the registrar about her request in the presence of the supervising consultant.

H Avoid conflict by agreeing to include the registrar on the abstract without doing so.

44. A ward clerk approaches you and asks whether you would look at a lump on his neck.

Rank in order the following actions in response to this situation (1 = Most appropriate; 5 = Least appropriate)

A Complete a cursory examination, before directing the ward clerk to a specialist.

B Complete a full examination with a chaperone in a side room.

C Direct the ward clerk to their GP.

D Book the ward clerk in for an ultrasound scan.

E Refuse.

45. Your FY1 colleague has decided to participate in a social media campaign highlighting rising waiting times for hospital discharge. In doing so, you offer some advice.

Choose the THREE most appropriate actions to take in this situation

A Identify patients by their bed numbers, instead of by name.

B Only cite specific examples that were in your previous rotation.

C Convey feelings of your whole department, not just your own, on the issue.

D Highlight personnel from other departments who might be responsible for the situation.

E Invite named colleagues from A&E and management departments to participate.

F Reflect on your rotations and offer your own professional experiences.

G Do not get involved in any social media campaign, as you will likely be in breach of your hospital contract.

H Contact your MP.

46. You are asked by the ward clerk to check the results of their recent biopsy.

Rank in order the following actions in response to this situation (1 = Most appropriate; 5 = Least appropriate)

A Print off the report.

B Suggest the ward clerk to speak with the referring doctor.

C Report the ward clerk to their line manager.

D Provide the results of the biopsy if they are normal, but otherwise refuse.

E Phone the referring team to ask if the results can be divulged.

ANSWERS

1. **C, B, D, A, E**

Confidentiality is important for maintaining patient dignity and trust in the medical profession. The security of a patient list cannot be guaranteed at home and most Trusts will have policies preventing staff from removing details in this form. The best answer is to raise the issue informally with your colleague (C)—this deals with the issue immediately and gives them an opportunity to reflect on their behaviour. Asking for a confidential waste bin (B) also deals with the problem, but less immediately, and does not guarantee that it will be used by this colleague. Speaking to your consultant (D) also addresses the problem indirectly, but it is less ideal than (B) because it risks jeopardizing your working relationship and may represent premature escalation. (A) is the first incorrect answer as this would appear childish, unnecessarily competitive, and misses the real concern about breaching patient confidentiality. The worst answer is (E) as duplicating your colleague's error only doubles the risk of a patient list being lost.

2. **E, B, D, C, A**

This is a difficult question. (E) is probably the best answer as you should already be doing everything in your power to maintain patient confidentiality, particularly information that is very sensitive. (B) is almost as good an answer as you are acting positively to respect your patient's request. It is not as good as (E) only because you should already have been doing everything possible to ensure information is secure. (D) is the first wrong answer for two reasons. First, you would not usually tell a patient they must talk to their family about a sensitive diagnosis outside the unique circumstance of there being a sexual partner at risk of infection. Second, although you cannot guarantee they will never become aware of his diagnosis, you should be able to confidently state that everything you do will protect his confidentiality. (C) is wrong as it breaches your patient's confidentiality unnecessarily. Some Trusts will have a system of indicating high-risk patients (e.g. coloured stickers), so phlebotomy staff can take additional precautions. However, there is an argument that maximal precautions should always be undertaken for invasive procedures and therefore this information would be unnecessary to share. In this case, writing 'HIV+' is incorrect as high-risk patients can be identified without disclosing their precise diagnosis. The worst answer is (A) because obscuring the diagnosis from his notes will mislead others and potentially place the patient at risk.

3. **A, C, D, E, B**

This group is exposing patient confidentiality to significant risk. The best answers are (A) and (C) as they address the problem contemporaneously and stand the best chance of protecting patient confidentiality. It is difficult to differentiate between the two, but you are likely to have more success speaking to an individual (A) than approaching the whole group (C). (D) would also address the problem but is less ideal because it does not stop the problem at the time it was occurring. However, you might not feel confident reprimanding colleagues on your own out of hours in a social environment and, in which case, you should raise the issue formally with the Trust (D). (E) is the first wrong answer as you have a professional duty to protect patients and challenge inappropriate behaviour. Some people might argue that (B) is at least an attempt to address the situation; however hospital security would likely be surprised by such a call and have no jurisdiction away from the hospital site.

4. **A, B, C, E, D**

You have a duty to take appropriate action following any concerns about patient care, dignity, or safety. The question raises the issue of verbal abuse by a member of staff against a vulnerable patient. (A) is the best answer because it addresses the issue immediately and separates the (potentially abusive) staff member from the patient. (B) is the first incorrect answer, even though a senior nurse is exactly the right person to speak to. This is because waiting for such a person introduces delay and does not ensure the immediate safety of this patient. (C) is also wrong because it introduces delay but, this time, you are speaking to the wrong people and risk prejudicing a disciplinary (or even criminal) investigation at a later time. However, (C) does imply that you are planning to take further action, even if it is not your role to investigate at this stage. (E) is not as good an answer as there is nothing in the question that justifies raising concerns externally when internal procedures are likely to be more expedient. (D) is obviously the worst answer as the GMC imposes a *duty* on doctors to raise concerns about patient dignity being compromised. You are not at liberty to ignore this event.

5. **C, E, B, D, A**

The GMC is clear that doctors must not sign contracts that fetter their ability to raise concerns. The simplest approach would be to politely explain that you are unable to sign such a document (C) as this might resolve the issue and could even prompt the Trust to avoid asking doctors to do this in future. An alternative, but more complicated, approach would be to contact the GMC or the medical defence organization for advice (E). The first incorrect answer is (B) as this ignores your new employer's improper attitude to whistleblowing and has a flavour of dishonesty as you are deliberately not returning the form in the hope that no one will notice. (D) is worse than (B) in that it is essentially the same, but this time you have deliberately agreed to something with which you have no intention of fulfilling. The worst answer is (A) as this is contrary to your professional obligation to raise concerns.

6. **C, A, B, D, E**

Although the diagnosis might be clear, you are responsible for the appropriateness of prescriptions. The best answer is therefore (C) as the patient will receive the correct treatment and you can ensure (for example) that they are not grossly unwell and have no allergies etc. (A) is the second best answer as the patient receives the correct treatment and you are working positively with your nursing colleague. You will commonly see this scenario played out on the wards; however, the responsible doctor should really assess their patient before prescribing. (B) is less ideal because, although it *may* be an appropriate treatment, antibiotic policies will reflect local resistance patterns and should be followed, unless there are good clinical reasons to depart from the protocol. (D) is the first obviously wrong answer as you are unlikely to provoke a positive reaction and have not treated the patient, and there is no reason why a nurse should not proactively identify clinical problems. (E) is the worst answer as it exposes the patient to significant harm by waiting for them to become compromised by their infection.

7. A, B, E, D, C

(A) is the correct answer as it is the most appropriate way of escalating concerns when other appropriate people have been unable to help. (B) is vital as it may protect you later and provides a valuable record; however, it does not in itself address the issue at hand. The other three answers are incorrect. Although carrying on and ignoring the problem is wrong (E), your part is at least neutral and others may highlight concerns instead. This makes (E) slightly better than (C) and (D) as these answers require you to actively breach patient confidentiality without any attempt to raise concerns internally first. (C) is the worst option only because a video record feels like a greater breach of privacy and there is an element of dishonesty in concealing a camera at work.

8. B, C, A, D, E

The two possible correct answers are (B) and (C). (B) is slightly better as you are proactively trying to attend a useful educational event while following your department's rules. (A) is the first incorrect answer as informal arrangements of this kind can breach departmental procedures and problems could arise, for example if that team member is deployed elsewhere because of staff shortages or is unwell on the day in question. However, you have at least made an effort to ensure your patients are looked after and that your clinical team (SHO and consultant) agree to your absence. (D) and (E) are both wrong as you are not entitled to attend and have made no effort to arrange clinical cover. However, (E) is worse because, on top of everything else, it means taking time away when you are being paid to be at work.

9. C, D, B, A, E

The best answer is clearly to do what you can to clarify misunderstandings (C) as this will help you understand the concerns and might facilitate a speedy resolution. (D) is the next best answer as making colleagues aware might help resolve issues and will keep them informed. (B) is also appropriate as PALS can offer advice independently of the clinical team and help this relative take her complaint further. However, she might not visit PALS after your conversation *and* (B) is not as good as (D) because the Ward Sister might be able to allay concerns or solve problems more expediently. (A) is the first wrong answer because you should never discourage others from exercising their right to complain about poor care. However, (E) is wrong for two reasons as it is unprofessional to complain about colleagues to third parties and, as in (A), you are attempting to influence the relative's decision about whether to complain.

10. **A, E, D, C, B**

Your first priority is Tim's safety. (A) is therefore the best answer because it ensures the drug is not administered. (E) is partially correct because it ensures the patient is safe, but it does not follow through to understand the cause of the error or to ensure it does not happen again. (D) is correct and should happen although in itself is insufficient to ensure the drug is not administered. The last two answers (C) and (B) address the cause of the mistaken prescription but fail to correct the immediate risk of an avoidable anaphylactic reaction. Raising the issue directly with the registrar (C) is better as it ensures immediate feedback (while they remember the case) and you can be satisfied yourself that feedback has been delivered. (B) would complete your clinical governance obligation to ensure errors are reported centrally to permit root cause analysis and identification of structural problems. However, as an isolated intervention, it is less important than the others.

11. **C, E, H**

This is a difficult question that implies a long-standing, cultural issue within your department, which you have interpreted as resulting in a lack of senior staff available to patients. It is difficult to know under the circumstances who best to contact, although, in such cases of uncertainty, the GMC suggests getting advice from a senior member of staff (H), a GMC employer liaison adviser (E), a medical defence organization (C), or Public Concern at Work, which is a charity providing confidential advice in such cases. The absent consultant (A), moonlighting SHO (G), and the consultant opposed to private practice (F) seem unlikely sources of impartial advice. Your partner (B) and friend from school (D) are not recommended as they might not understand the issues and/or are not bound by professional duty (e.g. to keep your concerns in confidence).

12. **B, D, H**

All doctors should encourage a culture in which concerns can be raised openly. This is particularly important for medical students who must learn early on not to ignore concerns. However, you should seek to clarify any misunderstandings and mention that consent might have been obtained without the student being present (B). Ultimately, the student should raise this issue with the consultant (D) to ensure they are not complicit in examining patients inappropriately. If they have concerns, their medical school will have its own 'raising concerns' policy (H).

You should not advise the student to keep quiet about their concerns. Specific consent for examination by medical students cannot be implied by consent to any particular operation (F). Raising the concern anonymously (G) may be unhelpful, as misunderstandings cannot be clarified and neither can further details be gathered for the concern to be acted upon. The student may wish to contact his medical school (H) before escalating concerns up the Trust hierarchy.

13. **B, D, E**

As a doctor, you have a responsibility to maintain your clinical skills and learn from patients. It is important to make allowance for this despite routine clinical commitments (F). Educational opportunities should be recognized for their intrinsic value and not simply to gain work-based assessments (H). This case clearly raises an issue of consent that is impossible to obtain under the circumstances. However, you are unlikely to feel a ruptured AAA in a well patient, and a brief abdominal examination may be appropriate (D) (A). As a doctor, you are in a different position from medical students who cannot directly influence a patient's care (C). If you were to examine the patient, it might be appropriate to ask the senior clinician responsible for their care (E). However, calling the patient's relatives at a time when they are probably distraught is likely to be unhelpful (G). You should certainly identify this gap in your experience and read about aneurysms, whether or not you examine the patient (B).

14. **A, E, F**

Work-based assessments are only one means of developing your clinical skills as a doctor. You may wish to examine every patient formally as if you were being observed and assessed (F). You might also gain by presenting and/or discussing the case (A). In this instance, the 'helpful' SHO might agree to watch you examine the patient before completing the assessment (E). Delaying the patient's assessment or care for your benefit is unacceptable (G).

Nevertheless, it is important to recognize that senior doctors have other commitments and cannot always be available to teach. Reminding the medical registrar of their teaching responsibilities is unlikely to nurture a joyous teacher–student relationship (B). Although assessments can be difficult to obtain, each trainee is responsible for achieving a minimum number (H). You should resist offers from other doctors to complete work-based assessments if the criteria for these have not been satisfied (C) (D). These offers jeopardize the probity of senior doctors and may deprive you of opportunities for genuine feedback.

15. **A, D, E**

It is your responsibility to satisfy all mandatory requirements of the Foundation Programme. However, foundation doctors are a key part of the clinical team and your absence could impact negatively on patient care. Therefore, you should take steps to minimize the impact of your absence.

You should attend mandatory commitments (A), unless this compromises patient safety. However, to resolve a potential conflict in future, you should seek advice from your consultant (D). It should be possible for another member of your team (e.g. the SHO or registrar) to lead the ward round (E) in your absence, and you can update this person to facilitate continuity of patient care. Only extraordinary circumstances should cause you to miss teaching (C) (F). If you have to miss a mandatory training session (e.g. because of a clinical emergency), you should ensure that you catch up in other ways such as private study (G). Signing the attendance register dishonestly (B) or asking someone else to do so (H) raises significant probity issues.

16. A, F, H

Doctors have a duty to promote the education and development of junior colleagues. (A) is correct as it ensures you will be able to fulfil your ward obligations and that the students are not under-sold with regard to the teaching they receive. (F) is ideal because it helps both you and the students achieve your goals for the day. (H) is helpful as it will stimulate the students to think while ensuring you are in a position to correct any gaps in their knowledge.

Signing students' attendance forms before sending them away (B) deprives them of teaching and casts doubt on your own probity. (C) is incorrect because it implies dishonesty and prevents the students from being taught. A formal tutorial might be useful but, under these circumstances, might conflict with ward commitments (D). Similarly, frivolous conversation (E) will not benefit the students nor ensure you complete your work on the ward. You should not exploit students by asking them to spend significant amounts of time on routine tasks with limited educational value (G).

17. A, E, F

You must be open and honest while delivering feedback in a constructive and professional manner. Raising your concerns throughout the placement (A) (B) will allow the student to explain his behaviour (F) and adjust his attitude. It would be dishonest to mark the student as 'satisfactory' in a domain if you actually believe otherwise (C). Instead, you should raise your concerns using specific examples (E), as when giving any negative feedback. However, concerns should only be raised with the Clinical Supervisor (D) or medical school (G) if their gravity warrants such interventions. Inciting the nursing staff to prejudge the incoming FY1 doctor (H) would be unhelpful and make it harder for him to change before starting the post.

18. C, D, F

Doctors must continue to develop knowledge throughout their careers and ensure that they are up-to-date. You should either ask for time during the day to complete the modules (C) or recognize their general benefit and do so at home (D). Refusing to comply with reasonable requests from your Trust (A) (E) (H) may cause employment difficulties.

Asking someone else to complete the modules (G) or doing so without reading their content (B) deprives them of their educational purpose. The former is also dishonest. Whether or not you found the modules helpful, you should consider providing feedback (F) so that they can be developed and improved for others.

19. C, D, G

You should avoid compromising your professional relationship with colleagues, including medical students (H). As a doctor on the team, you are responsible for their supervision, learning, and continued assessment. Attention should not be distributed unfairly (C) and romantic relationships should be discouraged (D), ideally at the earliest possible stage (G).

It would be unhelpful and unfair to avoid one particular student (A) and unprofessional to meet socially with ulterior motives (B). Although honesty is usually commendable, a frank discussion should be avoided (E) as it risks escalating the situation and surprising the student, particularly if you have misinterpreted their feelings. Similarly, asking questions of other students should be avoided (F).

20. B, F, H

There is no absolute rule preventing doctors from accepting gifts. However, the GMC does prohibit doctors from inviting or pressuring patients to make gifts, either to themselves or to anyone else. For this reason, you should not suggest that Sid donates money to a specific charity (G) or that he offers you a different amount (A).

Many Trusts will have policies on gifts (e.g. a maximum value) with which you should be familiar before accepting (H), and not afterwards (C). Although rules will vary, explaining that you are unable to accept the gift (B) is certainly an acceptable response. At the very least, you should not accept a high-value gift immediately without being convinced that it is more than a spontaneous gesture (F).

Transferring money from the patient to his daughter (E), when this was not his intention, would be inappropriate. Asking Sid to sign a statement (D) would overly formalize the situation and not protect you against the accusation of having coerced the gift. If you feel that this is necessary, given the gift's high value, this is an indicator that the gift is inappropriate.

21. C, D, F

In this dilemma, you must balance the principles of autonomy and non-maleficence. *Good Medical Practice* reminds us that 'doctors must not discriminate against patients by allowing personal views to adversely affect the professional relationship with patients or the treatment they provide' (A). The patient has severe postpartum haemorrhage (PPH) and a transfusion is indicated, but it cannot be given without consent. There is no risk to the life of the child (B). It is essential to confirm the patient's wishes and clarify with certainty any decision to refuse blood products (C) before ruling out a transfusion (D), and it should not be assumed that her wishes would be consistent with 'typical' Jehovah's Witnesses practice. It would be unethical to transfuse the patient without frank discussion while she remains conscious (E). In complex cases involving Jehovah's Witnesses, it is absolutely essential to involve senior colleagues, and a haematologist should also be involved early on (F). If the patient agrees to their involvement, a Hospital Liaison Committee for Jehovah's Witnesses can serve as a useful source of support for patients (G). There is no suggestion that the patient currently lacks the capacity to make a decision (H).

22. **B, D, A, E, C**

The correct answer is to perform a detailed physical examination and discuss this difficult situation with your senior (B). A less appropriate response would be to make the referral to the paediatric surgeon yourself without your senior's involvement (D). However, this would be better than ignoring your examination findings completely (A).

The assessment of a child's best interests must include the cultural/religious values of the child and/or parents. (E) is therefore an inappropriate referral, regardless of your own personal beliefs about religious circumcision, while (C) represents an even more serious accusation with greater implications for the parents. However, female genital circumcision (or mutilation) is a criminal offence and should be dealt with as such.

23. **E, D, C, B, A**

GMC guidance reminds us that probity is at the heart of medical professionalism. In this instance, it is important to address the issues of erroneous payment for locum shifts and working additional unpaid hours separately. The immediate priority should be to return any excess payment to your employer (E) before seeking to rectify your own excessive working hours, which may benefit from the input of your Educational Supervisor (D). (C) is not as good an answer, as completing a work diary in itself does not resolve the problem (although it may be necessary at some stage). The two wrong answers are (A) and (B), and there is little additional virtue to be found for donating your ill-gotten gains to charity. Even if it became evident that you had worked a similar number of hours unpaid, failure to raise the issue would cast serious doubt on your professional judgement. It could also lead to disciplinary, or even legal, action.

24. **B, D, F**

This scenario tests honesty about experiences and qualifications when applying for posts. The GMC requires that relevant information must not be deliberately omitted. While it is possible to mislead the reader with sentences that imply particular experiences (e.g. theatre exposure (A) (E) and courses attended (G)), it would be more honest to describe actual experiences on the ward (B) and alternative means of learning about operations (D), and to share your enthusiasm for future training (F). Arguments about too few opportunities (C) or unjustified claims of superior clinical competence (H) are unlikely to impress a selection panel.

25. C, E, B, A, D

Integrity is an essential foundation for any clinical or scientific study, including audit, which rests on the honesty and openness of the investigators. Conclusions must not be reached hastily from findings which may be misinterpreted. In this scenario, the best answer would be to discuss your concerns as soon as they arise with the consultant in question (C). She might be able to give a simple explanation (e.g. atypical case mix) and point you in the right direction for further data collection. This also addresses any potential issue early in case there is a short-term change that the consultant would like to implement. Although (E) raises your concerns from the audit and is very likely to show that there is no problem, it does introduce an unnecessary delay and is therefore worse than (C). (B) carries the same delay and is an inappropriate forum in which to raise this issue, but still offers the opportunity to address the underlying problems. However, raising the issue internally with the consultants in your department should be favoured in the first instance over contacting an external body (A); there is nothing in the question that would suggest this is necessary. The worst answer is (D), as you are potentially complicit in a cover-up.

26. D, F, H

The GMC sets out professional standards which guide undergraduate medical students (A). Behaviour outside the clinical environment can impact on a student's fitness to practise and should always justify public trust in the medical profession. The students should be asked to explain their actions (A). It is unlikely to be resolved at the time of the incident (B) and is not the responsibility of your own supervisors (C). Instead, the students should be confronted soon after the incident (F) (G) and their supervisors informed of this breach of professional duty (D). Informing your colleagues is unlikely to improve the situation (H). The police will deal with the students in their own way—your responsibilities as a member of the medical profession are different (E).

27. D, E, C, B, A

According to *Good Medical Practice*, doctors must inform the GMC *without delay* if they have 'accepted a caution or been charged or found guilty of a criminal offence anywhere in the world'. This includes motoring offences unless these are resolved by a fixed penalty notice. For this reason, (D) is the best answer. Asking your consultant for advice at the earliest opportunity should help signpost you to the correct procedure and is at least an attempt to transparency (E). Seeking independent advice is always helpful but does not go any distance towards discharging your responsibility as a professional to declare your caution abroad (C). (A) and (B) are clearly wrong as it is contrary to guidelines to delay informing the GMC. (A) is worse only because it implies indefinite dishonesty, rather than inappropriate delay (B).

28. **C, E, D, A, B**

Punctuality is an essential attribute for facilitating expeditious patient care. In this instance, a delay in printing the patient list has limited the time available to review each patient. None of the options is ideal and the question requires you to balance the practicalities of running an efficient ward round with the difficulties you are currently facing. In this instance, the best answer is to ask the medical student (if they are willing) to catch you up with the list once it is printed (C). This would allow the round to begin without delaying your consultant's list. (E) ensures that the list is available, but at the cost of a delayed endoscopy list and/or rushing the end of the ward round. (D) is less suitable as it risks missing patients on the ward round who might then be deprived of the opportunity to be assessed by a senior doctor. The two wrong answers are (A) and (B). (A) is unhelpful and is unlikely to endear you to your consultant, though it is otherwise a fairly neutral action. (B) by contrast is the worst answer as it is never appropriate to use personal email addresses to send patient information.

29. **D, B, A, E, C**

It is very tempting when answering these questions to latch on to a single algorithm for answering similar situations. For example, most scenarios are best answered by directly approaching the person about whom you are concerned first. This might even be the correct answer here, depending on your existing relationship with the FY1 doctor. However, in this case, the issue that has arisen is between a nurse and another doctor, and you are only involved as a bystander. It might then be more appropriate to report the concerning behaviour you have witnessed to an appropriate senior colleague and allow them to manage the situation from this point forth. For this reason, (D) is the best answer. The next best option *is* to contact the FY1 doctor directly and mediate between the two parties (B). Although this might resolve the current issue (B), it is not as good as (D) because only their Educational Supervisor will have an overall view of whether this represents a pattern of concerning behaviour. (A) is half-correct as the nurse probably should contact his line manager, but it sounds dismissive and unsupportive, and ignores the fact that you are a witness to 'bullying' behaviour at work. (E) does not really achieve anything as it is an impersonal means of communication and does not take the issue any further. Although elements of (C) appear correct, it is the worst answer only because you should never discourage a colleague from expressing their concerns.

30. **B, E, C, D, A**

It might be tempting to choose (E) as a way of recognizing your own limitations and seeking help early; however, the in-flight emergency *might* be something you are able to manage. A further call before even a cursory assessment of the patient would be excessive. You will often encounter this in the hospital, when you are asked to attend an emergency, and it is usually more appropriate to assess a patient yourself (even if briefly) before seeking further help, as there are often simple things you can do first, and assessing the patient helps guide the type of help that you ask for. For this reason, (B) is narrowly a better answer than (E). (C) is inappropriate as it implies a cursory examination and that you might not formally assess the patient in an effort to remain unidentifiable. However, it at least supposes that you are offering your assistance. (D) and (A) are incorrect answers as the GMC requires that 'in an emergency, wherever it arises, you must offer assistance, taking account of your own safety, competence, and the availability of other options for care'. (D) risks delaying review or treatment of a patient in extremis, whereas (A) supposes not offering your assistance at all. Although you should always work within your limits, inexperience is a poor reason for failing to act appropriately in an emergency.

31. C, E, D, B, A

Doctors must be willing to teach and train students and other doctors as part of their responsibility for the care of patients now and in the future. This necessity requires the appropriate skills and attitudes of an effective teacher, one of which is effective planning.

Whether it was wise to do so, you have promised teaching these students in preparation for their respiratory exam. You will need to be honest and upfront that you have not prepared adequately for this (although this is not an option). For this reason, (C) is the best answer, as you are obliged to attempt to provide some value to the students. (E) represents an attempt at teaching; even if you are not contributing to their knowledge, you can at least try to identify gaps and help them revise. (D) is clearly not as good, as this is not what the students have identified as an imminent learning need. However, some teaching is better than none, and the students might still be grateful for an opportunity to learn about a subject with which you are comfortable and confident teaching. (B) is essentially no teaching (for now) which is worse than (E), as previously explained. The worst answer is blaming the students who kept their part of the bargain (A).

32. C, E, G

As a foundation doctor, you will experience many practices for the first time (B), and the safe management of patients should be paramount (A). You should use an ABCDE approach and ensure that all patients are stable before completing a more thorough assessment (C). You are ultimately responsible for your actions when assessing and treating any patient (E), while the consultant takes responsibility for your training and supervision (D). In introducing yourself to a patient or parents, you are clarifying your position within the team of doctors providing their care (G) (F). Your introduction does not require a detailed account of your training and experiences as this may unduly compromise the trust placed in your advice (H). However, it is important to remain honest and transparent if asked about your grade or experience by the patient's family.

33. **C, D, E, B, A**

References should be written honestly and objectively, particularly with respect to positions in healthcare which may place patients at risk if individuals are appointed incorrectly. (C) and (D) are therefore the most appropriate answers. (C) appears more constructive as it offers an alternative to yourself as a referee while implying that there are more experienced people available to help with this request. Of the three incorrect responses, (E) is best because it makes an attempt to objectively determine whether the student is coping with their current course of study to which they should be committed before embarking on a second. The last two answers are difficult to distinguish between. You should probably express your concerns to the student, but write a generally supportive reference (B), rather than sabotaging his application with a poor reference, particularly without giving him some indication that this would happen if you were to do as he asked (A).

34. **D, A, B, E, C**

The most important fact here is that you are not told the patient is in extremis, and therefore there is no clinical urgency to perform an examination. There are a number of considerations, including the welfare of a scared and vulnerable patient, your colleague's difficulties as an inexperienced male member of the team, and the complications around examining a patient who has been the alleged victim of a sexual assault. (D) is the best answer, as he should examine the patient only if a chaperone can be available, and his initial examination is likely to be limited (i.e. no internal examination until senior support is available). If there is any doubt, or a chaperone is not available, then (A) would be the correct answer, although less ideal as it makes little progress in the management of the patient. (B) is less good, and while credit might be given for performing any examination of the patient with a chaperone, examination by inspection alone offers little clinical value. Although it is common practice to use a female relative as a chaperone, in a particularly sensitive case, this is not appropriate, and it is not common practice to ask a chaperone to sign in the notes (E). (C) is clearly the worst answer because an inexperienced male doctor should not perform an intimate examination on a minor who has suffered alleged sexual assault, regardless of whether there is a chaperone!

35. **C, B, D, E, A**

Even as a more junior doctor, it is essential to realize the impact that your comments can have on your own hospital and more widely across the profession itself, particularly those made available in the public domain. The best answers are clearly the two in which you are not providing any meaningful comment for the reporter at this time, as you are unprepared and inexperienced. (C) is probably preferable to (B) because the Trust is unlikely to agree to an FY1 doctor providing an interview on this subject. Although the next three are incorrect, clearly the better two—(D) and (E)—are the ones in which general comments are made and you do not refer specifically to your department or your theories about this particular issue (A). (D) is better than (E) because you are unlikely to come across well complaining about the ignorance of the general public in the public domain.

36. B, A, C, E, D

None of the answers is particularly good. (B) is probably the best answer because it gives you an opportunity to find out more precisely where difficulties with teaching provision have arisen, without requiring additional resources from the postgraduate medical office. As the FY1 representative, you carry the (perhaps unenviable) burden of ensuring some change is made if necessary. Although a full review into teaching may be excessive, this is the only other option you are provided with in which FY1 doctors' views are taken into consideration (A). (C) is less good as an answer because it introduces unnecessary delay, although there might be strategic reasons for wanting to raise the issue later. (D) and (E) are both unhelpful; (D) is worse as it appears to mislead the committee by suggesting that you have consulted widely amongst FY1 doctors.

37. E, C, B, A, D

The GMC requires that you never encourage patients or their relatives to offer gifts that will directly or indirectly benefit you, and you should make reasonable efforts to dissuade them from such offers. For this reason, (E) is the best answer as it perfectly mirrors this advice. The second best answer is to seek impartial professional advice (e.g. from a medical defence organization) as you are unlikely to have experience of receiving high-value gifts (C). This is probably more appropriate than informing the Ward Sister, but doing so (B) is at least an attempt to seek advice and may lead you to be directed towards your Trust's policy on acceptance of gifts. Accepting the gift with no attempt to dissuade the relatives should be your last option, particularly given that it is high value (D). Although there is no role for informing the GMC about receiving a gift, regardless of its value (A), this is probably a safer answer than (D).

38. C, E, D, B, A

All qualified doctors have a legal obligation to sign cremation forms and cannot refuse on personal or religious objections to cremation (Cremation Acts 1902 and 1952). (C) is therefore the correct answer. You should probably advise your colleague that, if they are the only doctor who can sign the form, they should do so to avoid unnecessary delay and distress to relatives. (E) is less helpful but still correct, as you are not giving your colleague the full benefit of your medico-legal knowledge but have done the right thing in declining to sign a cremation form for a patient you do not know. (D) would be improper advice, as your colleague going away for this reason would be unprofessional and risk delay to funeral arrangements and consequent further distress to family members. (A) is the worst option as you are not legally entitled to complete a cremation document as you have not cared for the patient during their last illness. This means that encouraging your colleague to lie (B) falls between simple unprofessional behaviour (D) and illegality (A).

39. D, C, A, B, E

Although you are keen to attend the course, it would be wrong to subvert the process for allocating places. If your colleague is unable to attend the course, he should explain this to the coordinators. Therefore, you should ask whether they would agree to transfer the place to you from your colleague, which is why (D) is the best answer. The second best answer is (C), as refusing the offer would allow the place to be reallocated more equitably. (A), (B), and (E) are all incorrect; of these, (A) appears to be preferable as everyone is satisfied by the arrangement. (B) is next, as you are willing to take the place on the course without completing your part of the arrangement. The worst option is clearly (E) as this risks leaving the A&E department understaffed as well as betraying your colleague's trust.

40. D, B, A, C, E

Your NHS employer has allocated a set amount of work per employee and may not have accounted for additional tasks on the private ward. Your primary responsibility is for your *own* patients, and their care must not be compromised by acquiescence to inappropriate requests, even if driven by your consultant. The best answer is (D) as you should generally approach the person most likely to resolve the situation satisfactorily, who is the consultant in this case. Speaking to another consultant would be less ideal but may lead to her imparting wise advice for you to follow (B). (A), (C), and (E) are wrong answers. (A) is probably the best of these; although you are unlikely to be entitled to additional money for work done during additional time, asking your consultant is unlikely to cause significant harm to anything, except your dignity and career! Attempting to coerce the patient would be much worse (C). But failing to answer your bleep (even if you think it's from a ward for which you are not responsible) could result in harm to patients if you are uncontactable (E).

41. A, F, H

There are two possibilities explaining this scenario—either the consultant's interpretation is correct or there is a real difference in outcome that needs to be raised. It would be reasonable to check your analysis to see whether you can identify a mistake that could explain the difference (A). The option to include others experienced in research (F) is another sensible strategy to clarify your data analysis. (H) could lead to the identification of errors in your study design or would be an initial step towards raising your concern formally with senior colleagues. Ignoring the finding would be incorrect as it potentially exposes patients to harm (B). The other options (D) (E) (C) are all likely to result in conflict without necessarily addressing the concern at hand.

42. A, C, B, E, D

You should avoid prescribing medication for family members and friends in any informal capacity and so (A) is the best answer. (C) is a refusal of sorts as it indicates that you, personally, are unwilling to prescribe or at least uncertain as to whether the request is appropriate. (B) is incorrect but clearly more appropriate than signing the prescription without first-hand experience of the patient (E). (D) is the last answer as it is clearly both dishonest and unhelpful.

43. **C, D, G**

This raises an issue of probity and professionalism. The priority should be to clarify whether the registrar has fulfilled the criteria for author-ship (C). The details in the question stem suggest that this has not been the case and so the honest response would be to decline authorship (D). This may require discussion in the presence of a senior third party, e.g. the research supervisor (G). Agreeing to the registrar's request for anything other than meeting the minimum requirement for authorship would be dishonest (E) (F) (H). Discussing the matter with the registrar's Educational Supervisor may eventually achieve the same as discussing with your supervising consultant (G) but is less direct and probably an over-reaction. This scenario is not relevant to the normal function of an ethics department (A).

44. **C, A, E, B, D**

The principle here is that a thorough consultation is necessary to exclude any serious condition, which likely requires a full history and examin-ation in the context of having access to the patient's medical records. This is best achieved by the ward clerk's GP (C). Direct referral to a specialist would be sub-optimal and potentially a poor use of resources, but the ward clerk would at least then see another doctor in more for-mal setting (A). Point blank refusal may be the correct option in some respects but is likely to interfere with your working relationship in future (E). It also means missing an opportunity to point a colleague towards a legitimate source of help for what might turn out to be a significant symptom. A full examination (perhaps including a hunt for axillary and/ or inguinal lymph nodes) in a side room would appear to take your role further than is appropriate outside the usual doctor–patient setting (B). (D) would appear to take responsibility for the ward clerk's clinical pres-entation, when this really should be coordinated by someone else, e.g. their GP. Although experienced doctors sometimes conduct such 'corri-dor consultations' and request investigations for colleagues, this is widely accepted to be sub-optimal and is not a route upon which an FY1 doctor should embark.

45. **E, F, H**

You are (almost) as free to become involved in campaigning as any other individual (G). You should, however, be careful about disclosing patient information (A) (B) or being seen to be speaking on behalf of your employer (C). Similarly, any such campaigning would need to be balanced against the need to maintain good relations with colleagues (D). This does not prevent you from sharing your own reflections (F), inviting specific colleagues to share their views (E), or making representations through your Member of Parliament in the same way as any other constituent (H).

46. **B, E, A, D, C**

While the patient has a legal right to the data (A), it is far better for the patient to liaise with the referring doctor directly (B) or to obtain the correct context from the referring team (E). Option (D) is not helpful as you are at risk of not understanding the implications of a negative biopsy result without full context. The patient will also likely learn the result from interpreting such conditional behaviour. (C) is an unhelpful over-reaction.

Chapter 10

Coping with pressure

Introduction

The Foundation Programme is tough. New doctors have to cope with taking responsibility for patients for the first time and managing the logistical difficulties that inevitably face those working in a complex environment. They often have to balance multiple competing priorities. Perhaps computed tomography (CT) scans need to be requested by 9.30 a.m. if they are to be scheduled for the same day, Mrs A has chest pain, Mr B is an outlier on a distant ward and has become acutely short of breath, and Mr C's relatives are angry because they have been waiting to speak to a doctor for an hour. You are part-way through taking blood and have three bleeps to answer (all potentially important but conferring new tasks), and your consultant needs to complete the ward round before her clinic starts … This would not be a remarkable day by any means.

It can be difficult to balance these responsibilities and do so without cutting corners. Criticism is inevitable as it is rarely possible to keep everyone happy all of the time.

Questions within this section will explore your resilience and ability to work under pressure. Through your responses, you will need to demonstrate a willingness to remain flexible, manage ambiguity, and adapt to changing circumstances.

The ability to remain calm while handling stressful situations arising with patients, relatives, and colleagues is of the utmost importance. Problems must be resolved directly but may require a diplomatic approach to avoid conflict. It is therefore important to speak to others respectfully, seek help early on, and remain aware of your own limitations.

There is growing recognition that such pressures can have long-term health implications for junior doctors. You must be aware of threats to your own health, and the British Medical Association (BMA) has reiterated that you have a duty to ensure that your 'health problems do not affect patient care'. Informal (so-called 'corridor') consultations are discouraged, and *Good Medical Practice* (2013) is clear that 'you must, wherever possible avoid providing medical care to yourself'. The BMA also reminds doctors that they have a 'duty to take action if they become aware that a colleague's health is affecting patient care'. Questions about recognizing your own health problems—or those of colleagues—and mitigating any risk to patients may well appear under this domain.

You should always be conscious of your limits as an FY1 doctor. In general, you should not be consenting patients for operations, making complicated discharge decisions, giving drugs they do not understand, or managing critically ill patients without support from a senior doctor. You should not be doing these things, regardless of how much you feel pressured to do so by others.

In general terms, foundation doctors should not be responsible for obtaining consent for advanced procedures (e.g. operations) from patients. This is because they are unlikely to have the depth or experience and knowledge that is required to fully counsel patients about the risks, benefits, and any alternative treatments. However, the GMC accept that a foundation doctor may obtain consent from such a procedure if they are *supervised when doing so* and the more senior doctor has overall responsibility for the consent process. One advantage of this is that foundation doctors can begin to develop good consent practices as part of a structured learning opportunity. The doctor responsible for the procedure would, however, be available to answer any additional questions and to ensure that informed consent has truly been obtained.

The London Deanery has previously circulated a useful document that includes details of the tasks deemed appropriate and inappropriate for foundation doctors. The procedures that were identified as always requiring supervision when performed by a foundation doctor were pleural tube drainage, ascitic fluid drainage, sigmoidoscopy, central line insertion, and nasogastric tube insertion.

It is worth considering the following three principles before you begin the questions within this SJT domain:

- Regardless of how many demands are made on your time, you must prioritize to ensure that the most important tasks are completed first.
- Patients who are haemodynamically unstable are your first priority. Those in pain or distress are second. Routine tasks (e.g. discharge summaries) can wait until an appropriate moment.
- If you are not coping with your workload to the detriment of patients, you must summon assistance or attempt to delegate tasks. If help is not available, it should be escalated to a senior colleague.

References and further reading

British Medical Association (2010). *Ethical Responsibilities in Treating Doctors Who Are Patients*. http://www.gmc-uk.org/doctorswhoarepatientsjanuary2010.pdf_62126868.pdf

Health Education East of England (2013). *Obtaining Informed Consent by Doctors in Training*. https://heeoe.hee.nhs.uk/sites/default/files/1397055514_vpgb_obtaining_informed_consent_by_doctors_in_training_2.pdf

Questions

1. You are a new FY1 doctor in an orthopaedic team. The morning ward round is running late, and both your consultant and registrar need to go to theatre. One patient has yet to be consented for a hemi-arthroplasty after fracturing her hip. Your registrar tells you to make sure that she is consented in time to be second on the morning list.

Rank in order the following actions in response to this situation (1 = Most appropriate; 5 = Least appropriate)

A Consent the patient before doing any other jobs.

B Complete all urgent jobs arising from the ward round, and then consent the patient.

C Explain that you are not sufficiently experienced to consent patients for this operation.

D Ask an SHO from another team who can perform hip hemiarthroplasties to take consent.

E Agree to consent the patient and then ask experienced nurses to show you how to do this correctly.

2. You are the FY1 doctor on call for medicine. After seeing a patient with pancreatitis, you recall the need to take an arterial blood gas (ABG). Unfortunately your only experience of this procedure was on a model two years previously. You have never attempted to perform an ABG on a patient before and are not feeling confident about success.

Rank in order the following actions in response to this situation (1 = Most appropriate; 5 = Least appropriate)

A Call the duty medical registrar and ask them to supervise your first ABG.

B Ask another FY1 doctor who is available and more confident with procedures to help.

C Attempt the procedure but without warning the patient about your inexperience.

D Wait until the end of your shift and then hand the job over to the night team.

E Attempt the procedure twice after talking to the patient, and then ask for help if unsuccessful.

3. As the FY1 doctor on call, you are bleeped by the pathology laboratory about an abnormal blood result. They give you a value representing severe hypernatraemia. You do not recall very much about hypernatraemia and have never managed a patient with this problem before.

Rank in order the following actions in response to this situation (1 = Most appropriate; 5 = Least appropriate)

A Call the duty medical registrar and ask what to do.

B See the patient to check that they are well, and then call the duty medical registrar.

C Find a computer terminal and Google 'hypernatraemia' for inspiration.

D Consult hospital guidelines, either in paper form or online.

E Prescribe a loop diuretic such as furosemide.

4. You are on a busy surgical ward round. Your consultant tells you to order an urgent CT scan and make sure that it happens that morning. Although you make a note on your jobs list to do this, you do not think that there is a good reason for doing the scan.

Rank in order the following actions in response to this situation (1 = Most appropriate; 5 = Least appropriate)

A Ask the consultant what the scan is for.

B Tell the duty radiologist that you disagree with doing the scan but have been told that it is urgent.

C Explain to your consultant you cannot order the scan as you disagree that it is appropriate.

D Ask a colleague in your team whether they can explain why the CT scan is necessary.

E Book an ultrasound instead and then reconsider the CT scan later depending on its results.

5. Matron has raised an issue about a drug that you prescribed incorrectly. You prescribed a ten-times overdose which fortunately was spotted by a vigilant pharmacist and never administered. Nevertheless, a clinical incident form has been completed and Matron is going to contact your Educational Supervisor. You feel that this error was caused by being overly tired.

Rank in order the following actions in response to this situation (1 = Most appropriate; 5 = Least appropriate)

A Tell Matron that the error was not your fault because the Trust made you work unsafe hours.

B Accept personal responsibility, but explain the factors that you believe contributed to the error.

C Ask Matron not to contact your Educational Supervisor as this was an isolated error.

D Use your e-portfolio to record the error, and reflect on its reasons so as to avoid this happening again.

E Ask to meet your Educational Supervisor to discuss the error and your concerns about the night rota.

6. You are enjoying an evening meal with your friends when you remember ordering a blood test for an unwell patient, the result of which you forgot to check or hand over.

Rank in order the following actions in response to this situation (1 = Most appropriate; 5 = Least appropriate)

A Make a note to check the result first thing in the morning before the ward round.

B Call the duty FY1 doctor through the switchboard and ask them to check the result.

C Put the issue out of your mind—it is important to 'turn off' after work.

D Reflect on how this test was missed and resolve to develop a system to ensure that such an error does not occur in the future.

E Drive back to the hospital to check the result yourself.

7. An FY1 doctor with whom you work closely says she is concerned that you seem 'down' and have been so for a few weeks. You have noticed that your mood is lower than normal but put this down to stress and tiredness. You do not think that you are clinically depressed and are embarrassed by your colleague raising the possibility.

Rank in order the following actions in response to this situation (1 = Most appropriate; 5 = Least appropriate)

A Clarify the nature and reasons for your colleague's concern.

B See your Educational Supervisor at the next possible opportunity to discuss your mental health.

C Make a routine appointment with your GP.

D Ask other FY1 colleagues whether they think you are depressed.

E Use a depression screening tool to determine whether you require drug treatment.

8. After an emergency operation, a patient is left with a colostomy. You are the first doctor to see the patient once he becomes conversant, and he asks whether the bag is permanent. You are certain that colostomies can be reversed but do not remember very much else.

Rank in order the following actions in response to this situation (1 = Most appropriate; 5 = Least appropriate)

A Tell the patient that his colostomy will be reversed.

B Explain that you are an FY1 doctor and cannot answer complicated surgical questions.

C Explain that colostomies can sometimes be reversed and that you will help find out the plan in his case.

D Offer to ask your registrar to drop by later on to answer specific questions.

E Put time aside to read about stomas so you can answer questions more fully next time.

9. You are seeing a very unwell patient on your ward. He is complaining of chest pain and is also becoming increasingly hypotensive, despite fluid resuscitation. Over the previous few minutes, he has started to become drowsy. Although you are an FY1 doctor, you recently completed an Advanced Life Support (ALS) course and feel confident in managing acutely unwell patients.

Rank in order the following actions in response to this situation (1 = Most appropriate; 5 = Least appropriate)

A Summon the resuscitation team.

B Continue to manage the patient, regardless of their clinical condition.

C Call the consultant on his mobile phone.

D Call the SHO on her mobile phone for advice.

E Continue managing the patient unless he continues to deteriorate.

10. Your consultant asks you to meet her in her office. She tells you that she is concerned about your performance, specifically that you sometimes arrive late for her ward rounds and that your level of clinical knowledge is below her expectations of a doctor at your level. You disagree with this assessment, as you have only been late twice and do not think that there are any particular gaps in your knowledge.

Rank in order the following actions in response to this situation (1 = Most appropriate; 5 = Least appropriate)

A Explain why you feel that her assessment is unfair, and ask her to provide specific examples to illustrate her concerns.

B Ask the foundation school about the possibility of changing consultants as there has been a relationship breakdown.

C Ask the consultant for advice about how you can act on her concerns and improve your performance.

D Using your e-portfolio, conduct a Team Assessment of Behaviour (TAB) round looking for evidence of concern about your performance from other colleagues.

E Tell the consultant that you believe your knowledge to be no worse than that of other FY1 doctors and that you won several prizes at medical school.

11. You have always enjoyed alcohol but recently have been drinking more than usual. There is no reason for you to think that this has affected your performance and you have never been drunk at work. However, a number of junior colleagues have commented on your alcohol intake, and one has told you that she is concerned that you are developing a dependency. As a result, you have begun to worry about your intake.

Choose the THREE most appropriate actions to take in this situation

A Ask a friend with whom you socialize whether he/she thinks that you are drinking too much.

B Ask other FY1 doctors not to joke about your drinking, as you feel that this undermines your professional reputation.

C Use a validated assessment tool (e.g. CAGE) to determine whether you have developed an alcohol problem.

D Make an appointment with your GP to discuss your concerns about your alcohol intake.

E Discuss the issue with your Educational Supervisor at your next meeting.

F Stop drinking for a week to see if you develop withdrawal symptoms.

G Think carefully about your reasons for drinking more than usual recently, and consider modifying your drinking pattern.

H Stop going out with colleagues, and drink secretly instead to avoid damage to your reputation.

12. You have been working as an FY1 doctor for six weeks but struggle with intravenous cannulation; in fact, you have yet to site one successfully despite several attempts. You are concerned about the distress caused to patients by your unsuccessful attempts, and your inability to cannulate is starting to have an impact on the length of your working day.

Choose the THREE most appropriate actions to take in this situation

A Ask colleagues to site intravenous cannulae as often as possible until your ability improves.

B Using your e-portfolio, reflect on what it is that you are finding difficult about intravenous cannulation and how you can overcome this.

C Ask a senior colleague to supervise a series of cannulation attempts.

D Avoid trying to cannulate patients with 'difficult veins', and ask colleagues to see them instead.

E Consider modifying career aspirations to specialties that are less procedural.

F Continue to practise, recognizing that the procedure will become easier as you do.

G Attempt to cannulate each patient no more than once; if unsuccessful, bleep the duty anaesthetist for assistance.

H Tell every patient that they have 'difficult veins' so that their expectations of success are set low from the outset.

13. You are a lone FY1 doctor seeing an elderly patient on the ward who is hypotensive despite being given intravenous fluids. You are concerned that the only intervention you know for managing hypotension has not worked in this case.

Choose the THREE most appropriate actions to take in this situation

A Ensure that the patient has a valid Not For Resuscitation order in case they suffer a cardiac arrest.

B Accept that the patient is normally hypotensive and avoid further intravenous fluids.

C Call your SHO or other senior doctor for advice and assistance.

D Ask the nursing staff to put out a peri-arrest call.

E Begin administering inotropes if further fluid challenges fail to increase the blood pressure.

F Ask the patient's family to attend as their relative is probably dying.

G Ensure that you have good intravenous access and give another fluid challenge.

H Monitor the patient carefully for signs of deterioration.

14. You are feeling stressed as the on-call FY1 doctor and have just found yourself becoming angry with two sets of relatives in quick succession.

Choose the THREE most appropriate actions to take in this situation

A Take a short break to regain perspective.

B Ask a colleague to help share your workload if they are able to.

C Resolve not to speak with any more relatives on this shift as your priority must be unwell patients.

D Apologize to the relatives so that they are unlikely to complain.

E Consider what factors led to the altercations and address these as far as possible.

F Ask security or a nursing sister to remove the relatives so that you are not interrupted again.

G Manage your frustration by berating a medical student because he is unable to cannulate a patient.

H Check the time—it may be nearly time to go home.

15. Your manager emails to say that a written complaint has been received about your management of a patient seen in A&E. This concerns a patient whom you saw after a fall, but you did not document a proper examination. A fractured hip was missed for 72 hours.

Choose the THREE most appropriate actions to take in this situation

A Edit the notes to include features that you honestly recall at the time persuaded you that the patient did not have a broken hip.

B Edit the notes to include features that were not present but might make your mistake easier to forgive.

C Submit a factual description of events within the deadline imposed.

D Think honestly about the case and what you would do differently in future.

E Ignore the email as you are rotating to a new hospital next week.

F Explain that you were very busy that day and could not thoroughly examine every patient.

G Document your formal response and ask to be informed of the outcome of this complaint.

H Submit a response whenever you are able to—the clinical care of your current patients comes first.

16. Your consultant calls to ask you to relocate a dislocated total hip replacement for a patient on the orthopaedic ward. He mentions that you should give intravenous sedation first. When you tell him that you have never sedated a patient before, he tells you to use propofol and ketamine, and then hangs up the phone.

Choose the THREE most appropriate actions to take in this situation

A Call the consultant back to clarify what doses you should use and what movements are necessary to replace the dislocated limb.

B Call the consultant back to say that you are unwilling to do as he asks.

C Use the *British National Formulary* to determine doses.

D Sedate the patient and then find the duty orthopaedic registrar if you are unable to relocate the dislocated hip.

E Contact your Educational Supervisor at the first possible opportunity to discuss this request.

F Contact another senior orthopaedic colleague if your consultant does not answer or offers no further advice.

G Attempt to relocate the hip without using sedation.

H Sedate the patient and attempt to relocate the hip.

17. A patient asks you why you are ordering a CT scan to eliminate stroke as a possible cause of her symptoms. She is worried about radiation risk and wants a magnetic resonance imaging (MRI) scan instead. You do not recall precisely why CT is used as the first-line investigation for stroke.

Choose the THREE most appropriate actions to take in this situation

A Tell her that CT is probably cheaper than MRI.

B Explain that you are a junior doctor and cannot answer questions about complex investigations.

C Call the duty radiologist and hand the phone to the patient so that they can have an informed discussion.

D Explain that you do not know the answer but will speak with someone to find out the reason.

E Carefully explain the risks and benefits of having a CT scan, looking up information first if you are uncertain.

F Tell her that she cannot have an MRI scan and clearly document that she refused the CT scan.

G Ask your consultant to visit on his ward round the following week to discuss management options.

H Use this question to identify a gap in your knowledge and read around the subject during a spare moment.

18. Your registrar suggests one morning before the ward round that your appearance is inappropriate. In particular, he says that you are showing too much of your chest and are wearing a watch.

Choose the THREE most appropriate actions to take in this situation

A Remove the watch immediately as it conflicts with Trust policy.

B Explain that you had not realized that your dress was inappropriate and will consider this before coming to work the next day.

C Point out that your consultant also wears a watch.

D Wear more revealing clothes the following day to show you are free to interpret the Trust dress code yourself.

E Tell your registrar that he should be more interested in your clinical ability than your choice of clothes.

F Decline to participate in the ward round because you have been insulted by the registrar.

G Tell your consultant that your registrar was insulting and bullying before the ward round.

H Seek feedback from other colleagues if you are uncertain whether your clothes really are inappropriate.

19. You are on call at night and have not eaten since coming to work. You are very tired and can feel yourself nodding off to sleep within a few seconds of sitting down. You are about to break away for a sandwich when a Ward Sister asks you to write two drug charts for patients who have just been admitted.

Choose the THREE most appropriate actions to take in this situation

A Explain that you were planning to go for a break.

B Offer to write the drug charts later on.

C Explain that writing drug charts is not a job for the on-call doctor and is best left to the ordinary ward team instead.

D Have a quick look, prescribe any urgent drugs, and then go for your sandwich.

E Ask the nurse to complete the drug chart for you to sign when you get back.

F Ask how urgent the drugs are and use this information to prioritize the task.

G Tell the nurse that she should not bother you for such a routine task.

H Complete the drug charts as requested.

20. You know that you do not always communicate well when feeling stressed and want to avoid this impacting on your relationship with colleagues.

Choose the THREE most appropriate actions to take in this situation

A Use Team Assessment of Behaviour (TAB) rounds and informal feedback from colleagues to gauge your success at managing stress.

B Tell other team members early on that they should avoid making you stressed.

C Ask other FY1 doctors on your team to be responsible for shared tasks to minimize your workload.

D Make sure that you always go home at five o'clock.

E Try to streamline your work effectively so that you are not left with lots of tasks to complete at the end of the day.

F Talk to senior colleagues early if you think that the workload is getting on top of you.

G Drink alcohol in the evenings to 'loosen up'.

H Ask Human Resources (HR) for time each week to attend yoga and relaxation classes.

21. As the on-call FY1 doctor, you should finish at 10 p.m. and then hand over to the night SHO. However, one particular SHO refuses to accept jobs that he feels should have been completed during your shift. As a result, you find yourself leaving at 1 a.m. whenever he is scheduled to work nights.

Rank in order the following actions in response to this situation (1 = Most appropriate; 5 = Least appropriate)

A Document that the SHO refused to accept a handover and then go home.

B Stay late if necessary to ensure that patient safety is not compromised.

C Raise the issue with an appropriate person (e.g. your Educational Supervisor or line manager) as a priority on the following day.

D Report the night SHO to the GMC.

E Explain that you have completed as many tasks as you were able to and that he should assume responsibility for them at the end of your shift.

22. You are a surgical FY1 doctor expected to be prepared in advance of the morning ward round at 7.30 a.m. Your Clinical Supervisor tells you from the outset that you must also attend the 8 p.m. evening ward round. These hours conflict with the 9 a.m. to 5 p.m. working pattern indicated by your contract.

Rank in order the following actions in response to this situation (1 = Most appropriate; 5 = Least appropriate)

A Remind your consultant that you are contracted to work between 9 a.m. and 5 p.m.

B Slip off home for a few hours each day to remain compliant with the European Working Time Directive.

C Ignore your consultant's instructions and work from 9 a.m. to 5 p.m. as you are required to do.

D Accept that long hours are an inevitable part of any surgical post.

E Seek advice from your Educational Supervisor.

23. Your registrar calls you during the day and tells you that a patient's suprapubic catheter has fallen out and needs to be reinserted. You explain that you have never done this before, but he says that it is simple and that no one else is free to help until the operating list finishes eight hours later. He is insistent.

Rank in order the following actions in response to this situation (1 = Most appropriate; 5 = Least appropriate)

A Politely explain that you cannot perform the procedure safely and will need supervision.

B Ask another doctor with relevant experience to assist.

C Read about the procedure before having a go.

D Do as you are told, but document carefully that you were acting under your registrar's instructions.

E Refuse to help as you are inundated with other ward jobs.

24. An elderly patient with pneumonia is deteriorating despite antibiotic treatment. As the on-call medical FY1 doctor, you plan to discuss changing antibiotics with the duty consultant microbiologist. However, the nursing staff and patient's family are united in wanting treatment to be withdrawn to stop the patient from suffering. You seem to be alone in wanting to continue treating the patient aggressively.

Rank in order the following actions in response to this situation (1 = Most appropriate; 5 = Least appropriate)

A Familiarize yourself carefully with the case and try to understand why the family and nursing staff want to withdraw treatment.

B Insist on continuing with your plan as you are ultimately responsible for the patient.

C Stop all active treatment to hasten the patient's death and so end her discomfort.

D Contact a senior doctor to ask for their decision.

E Tell the patient's family to think carefully about the options and that you will do as they want if all members agree.

25. You are on call and bleeped by a ward nurse about a bag of blood that was mistakenly taken out of the fridge. As it cannot now be returned, she asks you to prescribe it for the patient so that it is not 'wasted'. You are not intending to visit the ward for some time and the nurse sounds frustrated as the blood will be lost 30 minutes after removal from the refrigerator.

Rank in order the following actions in response to this situation (1 = Most appropriate; 5 = Least appropriate)

A Go to the ward immediately to prescribe the blood.

B Tell her that you will not authorize a transfusion simply to avoid waste.

C Tell her that she should not have removed the bag unnecessarily and complete a clinical incident form after your shift.

D Encourage her to put the bag back in the refrigerator so that it can be returned to the blood bank for other patients.

E Explain that transfusion carries significant risks and there is no benefit in transfusing a non-anaemic patient.

26. An experienced staff nurse asks you to sign a prescription for a sleeping tablet that she administered an hour ago. You decline as this does not seem to be correct, but the Ward Sister says you have to sign as this is how things have always worked in their unit.

Rank in order the following actions in response to this situation (1 = Most appropriate; 5 = Least appropriate)

A Sign the prescription retrospectively.

B Tell both nurses that only doctors have the required training to decide which drugs to prescribe.

C Check the drug details to ensure that there were no contraindications and that an appropriate dose was administered.

D Advise that a note should be made on the prescription chart and hospital notes to indicate the drug was administered.

E Explain that an authorized prescriber must agree before drugs are given in future.

27. You are an FY1 doctor and part of the cardiac arrest team. On arriving at an arrest, you find that no one is managing the patient's airway despite a number of senior doctors being present. Other appropriate activities are taking place.

Rank in order the following actions in response to this situation (1 = Most appropriate; 5 = Least appropriate)

A Stand back so that you do not distract the arrest team leader.

B Ask the team leader why no one is managing the airway.

C Move to the patient's head and use airway adjuncts as appropriate.

D Ask whether an anaesthetist is present and, if not, whether they are on their way.

E Help with chest compressions because these are easily within your comfort zone.

28. The on-call bleep is constantly going off and you have a number of jobs to prioritize. You need to determine which to attend to first and then in order of priority.

Rank in order the following actions in response to this situation (1 = Most appropriate; 5 = Least appropriate)

A A 55-year-old man with central chest pain.

B An angry daughter who wants to discuss why her mother is developing bed sores and is threatening a formal complaint.

C A 40-year-old woman with metastatic cancer with bony pain needing analgesia review.

D A 24-year-old man after an elective orthopaedic operation who wants to go home but first needs a discharge summary and prescription.

E A 90-year-old woman with a pneumonia who is hypotensive and became unresponsive a few moments ago.

29. You are clerking patients in the Emergency Department. Your current patient is in police custody and, at the point of discharge, the accompanying officers ask you for a copy of the discharge summary. The patient asks you not to provide them with any details, but the officers insist that you *must* cooperate with their request.

Rank in order the following actions in response to this situation (1 = Most appropriate; 5 = Least appropriate)

A Politely explain to the police officers that you cannot provide information without your patient's consent.

B Discuss with a consultant if the officers insist.

C Give a discharge summary to the patient, knowing that it might be confiscated later on.

D Give the officers a discharge summary, as helping the police is in the public interest.

E Tell the officers that there are no circumstances under which you would betray your patient's confidence.

30. You are called from the private wing of your hospital. The receptionist there asks for a cannula to continue a blood transfusion that is half completed. She called the responsible consultant at home who told her to bleep the on-call FY1 doctor to resite the cannula.

Rank in order the following actions in response to this situation (1 = Most appropriate; 5 = Least appropriate)

A Decline to resite the cannula, regardless of the clinical situation and suggest that the consultant comes in from home to do so as it is his private patient.

B Assess the urgency of the transfusion and prioritize according to your other tasks.

C Help if you are able to, but let the receptionist know that they should have someone capable of cannulating patients on site.

D Cannulate the patient, but leave an invoice with the receptionist for £80.

E Contact a responsible person (e.g. the duty manager) to ask about the appropriateness of attending to tasks in the private wing.

31. You are on call and are approached by a staff nurse who admits to giving an unfamiliar drug stat instead of as an infusion over 12 hours. She asks you to see the patient but not to tell anyone about the error.

Choose the THREE most appropriate actions to take in this situation

A Review the patient as a priority.

B Call the duty manager immediately to request that the nurse be removed from work.

C Explain that you cannot cover up the error but that you will let her speak with the Ward Sister first.

D See the patient, but do not write in the notes to avoid causing the nurse career difficulties.

E Complete a formal incident form as soon as possible after the event.

F Call the intensive care registrar to discuss urgent transfer as the patient has been overdosed.

G Encourage the patient to vomit and prescribe intravenous fluids to flush out the drug.

H Tell the nurse that you cannot help but to bleep you if the patient deteriorates.

32. The daughter of an elderly patient asks you for an update about her mother's condition. A recent CT scan was suspicious of lung cancer and your patient has asked you not to tell anyone else to keep them from worrying. The daughter says she 'knows something is wrong' and it is unfair to keep the family 'in the dark'.

Choose the THREE most appropriate actions to take in this situation

A Empathize with the daughter, but explain that you cannot disclose this information without her mother's consent.

B Advise her you will call security if she persists in bothering you for information.

C Tell her that the CT scan was normal and that her mother will be discharged soon.

D Explain that her mother has asked you not to discuss certain aspects of her care with anyone.

E Tell her the results of the CT scan, but ask her not to tell the patient that you have done so.

F Discuss with your patient at the next opportunity to ensure that she understands the effect that withholding information might have on close family members.

G Talk openly with the daughter, as her mother is elderly and probably lacks capacity.

H Give her your consultant's mobile number so that she can discuss directly with your senior.

33. You are on call for medicine but are making no progress with your tasks because you are fielding so many bleeps. There are a number of acutely unwell patients on the wards awaiting assessment and the Emergency Department is now calling to inform you that patients are breaching.

Choose the THREE most appropriate actions to take in this situation

A Remove the batteries from your bleep and begin your existing tasks.

B Call your senior to let them know that you are not coping with the workload.

C Make a clear list of tasks in order of clinical priority.

D Explain to the Emergency Department that you have yet to assess potentially unwell patients and cannot assist for some time.

E Go to the Emergency Department, but document that this distracted you from other tasks in case anything goes wrong.

F Have a coffee break now as you work better when rested and are unlikely to get lunch later.

G Draft a letter to the Chief Executive complaining about the effect of your workload on patient care.

H Tell the Emergency Department that the Trust should appoint more doctors if it wants to avoid patient breaches.

34. You are experiencing relationship difficulties at home and this is affecting your ability to cope at work. The radiologist has just refused a CT request which your consultant said is very urgent and you burst into tears after leaving the radiology department.

Choose the THREE most appropriate actions to take in this situation

A Take a few minutes to compose yourself, and then alert your consultant to the radiology decision.

B Send an email to your team, explaining that you are very stressed and should be spared difficult tasks for the foreseeable future.

C Take a break and speak to a supportive colleague if possible.

D Go back and plead with the radiologist to accept your request.

E Contact the Medical Director to complain that the radiologist was obstructive.

F Tell Medical Staffing that you are unwell and have to go home to manage your domestic affairs.

G Ask another FY1 colleague to speak to the radiologist about your urgent CT request.

H Seek advice from your Educational Supervisor and/or Occupational Health if you continue to struggle at work.

35. You are a surgical house officer. The other FY1 doctor on your firm has called in sick and you feel that the workload is unmanageable for a single person. Your SHO apologizes for leaving you with so much to do but says that he 'has to go to theatre' or his logbook will suffer.

Choose the THREE most appropriate actions to take in this situation

A Tell the SHO that patient care should come before his logbook.

B Explain to the SHO that you cannot cope and need some help.

C Explain to the senior nurse on each ward that they should not bleep you unless patients are 'really sick'.

D Tell the SHO that you would like to go to theatre instead as he will be more efficient on the ward anyway.

E Ensure that your consultant or another senior doctor on the team knows that you are working alone.

F Call in sick tomorrow in case your colleague is away again and you are left alone for a second day.

G Carefully prioritize jobs and explain to the senior nurse on each ward that you are working alone and might be slower to respond than usual.

H Delay all patient discharges until the following day when your colleague might have returned.

36. You are ambushed leaving the ward by a group of relatives who are angry about the care of one of your patients who is now on the intensive therapy unit (ITU). They are asking lots of questions and one is videoing the interaction using a smart phone.

Choose the THREE most appropriate actions to take in this situation

A Say 'no comment' and block the camera with your hand.

B Try to ignore the camera and act as you would if it were not there.

C Explain that you are unable to talk about a patient's care without their permission.

D Tell the relatives that the Ward Sister is in a better position to answer their questions.

E Contact security if you feel threatened or their presence is obstructing your work.

F Answer questions to defuse the situation.

G Tell the group that you are from another team and have never heard of this particular patient.

H Try to confiscate the camera as you do not wish to be videoed.

37. You did not complete any alcohol screening questionnaires for patients admitted the previous week. A senior doctor tells you that this means that the Trust will lose a lot of money and that you should 'make up' answers to the questions retrospectively. You seek support from your consultant who tells you to do it to keep the Trust happy.

Choose the THREE most appropriate actions to take in this situation

A Decline to complete screening questionnaires dishonestly.

B Complete the questionnaires, as you have been told to do so by two senior colleagues.

C Contact a tabloid newspaper to report that Trusts are submitting false data for financial reward.

D Do not complete the questionnaires, but tell the senior doctor that you did so.

E Explain that you will make a particular effort to complete screening questionnaires the following week if these are important for the Trust.

F Refuse to complete the questionnaires, as they are unhelpful and interfere with patient care.

G Put the afternoon aside to call all discharged patients and complete the questionnaires by telephone interview.

H Explain that you realize the importance of the questionnaires to the Trust but that you do not think it is correct to complete the forms retrospectively.

38. A young patient with a pericardial effusion wants to leave hospital to attend his brother's wedding. Both the patient and his family plead with you to discharge him earlier than your consultant had initially planned, albeit without knowing his social circumstances. The patient appears to be very well and has normal observations.

Choose the THREE most appropriate actions to take in this situation

A Explain the risks of premature discharge, looking these up or seeking senior advice if you are uncertain.

B Tell the patient that your consultant's word is final and that he cannot leave earlier.

C Explain that the patient can self-discharge at any point if he wishes to do so.

D As the patient is haemodynamically stable, agree to discharge him earlier than planned.

E As the patient is haemodynamically stable, let him leave hospital for 24 hours to attend the wedding.

F Tell the patient that you will not stop him if he wants to go and that he can find the risks of pericardial effusion easily enough online.

G Tell the patient that his health should always come ahead of family engagements.

H Contact a senior doctor for advice.

39. You have finished a night shift and are exhausted. As you are preparing to go home, you receive a call from the day FY1 doctor to say they are suffering from diarrhoea and vomiting and cannot work as a consequence. You are due to work the following night as well.

Choose the THREE most appropriate actions to take in this situation

A Tell the FY1 doctor to pull himself together and come into work.

B Leave your bleep in a designated place.

C Let the site manager know that the day FY1 doctor is unable to come to the hospital.

D Head home as you have already worked a full night shift and are unsafe to continue working.

E Work as much of the day shift as you can, before you cannot continue and need to alert the responsible manager.

F Continue working to the best of your ability.

G Keep holding the bleep, but decline to review patients, as you are tired and unsafe.

H Ask the responsible manager to arrange appropriate cover so you have time for sufficient sleep before returning to work.

40. An elderly patient with known dementia is attempting to leave the ward. He has punched a healthcare assistant who tried to encourage him back to his bay. You do not believe that he has capacity to leave the ward.

Choose the THREE most appropriate actions to take in this situation

A Try to talk to the patient from a safe distance.

B Tackle the patient's legs and try to break his fall.

C Contact security urgently.

D Try to conduct an Abbreviated Mental Test Score (AMTS) examination from a safe distance.

E Attend to the healthcare assistant's injuries as soon as it is appropriate to do so.

F Shout and wave at the patient to encourage him back into the ward.

G Sedate the patient with propofol for his own safety and the safety of others.

H Continue with your work, as agitated patients are a problem for the nursing team.

41. You page the medical registrar for a third time, as you are worried about a sick patient you have been asked to review on a weekend on-call shift. Despite asking him to review your patient an hour ago, he still has not attended.

Rank in order the following actions in response to this situation (1 = Most appropriate; 5 = Least appropriate)

A Notify his Clinical Supervisor.

B Page him again.

C Call your consultant for advice.

D Document your attempted calls, do not alter your management plan, and check in again in one hour.

E Continue to manage as you see best, based on the new findings.

42. You are reviewing patients in A&E. A Muslim family requests only a female Muslim doctor treat their 17-year-old daughter.

Rank in order the following actions in response to this situation (1 = Most appropriate; 5 = Least appropriate)

A Try to accommodate the request if possible.

B Establish what their particular concerns are.

C Invite the hospital imam to speak with the family before reviewing the patient.

D Refuse any further treatment.

E Ask your consultant to speak with the patient.

43. You are finding it difficult to meet with your Educational Supervisor for one of your scheduled meetings, because of his commitments, which is now two months late.

Choose the THREE most appropriate actions to take in this situation

A Meet with his secretary.

B Ask your Clinical Supervisor for advice.

C Arrive unannounced at the end of his clinic.

D Inform the Postgraduate Dean.

E Email your supervisor with a copy to the Medical Director.

F Be patient, and accommodate last-minute changes, even if it means missing your meetings.

G Write your Educational Supervisor's comments on your progress report, so he can sign them quickly.

H Email the Educational Supervisor each day as a reminder.

44. You are on a GP placement and are seeing the same patient with swollen legs for the third time. Although you are confident about having excluded all serious causes, the patient is concerned that his symptom is caused by cancer.

Choose the THREE most appropriate actions to take in this situation

A Seek to explore the underlying anxieties.

B Arrange intensive investigations that you do not feel are objectively indicated.

C Pretend to perform a second re-examination.

D Invite the patient to return to see one of the experienced GPs.

E Make a hospital referral to a specialist.

F Seek inpatient admission for psychiatric assessment.

G Prescribe antidepressants.

H Re-emphasize your assessment that there is not a sinister cause.

45. You discharge a patient from A&E, who asks you for money for a taxi home. He cannot arrange his own transportation until the following day.

Rank in order the following actions in response to this situation (1 = Most appropriate; 5 = Least appropriate)

A Consult the nurse in charge.

B Offer him the money if you can.

C Suggest he remains as an inpatient for pain management until the morning.

D Inform the vulnerable adult protection team.

E Refuse.

ANSWERS

1. **C, D, E, A, B**

GMC guidance states that the doctor providing treatment (i.e. the operation in this example) is responsible for obtaining informed consent. He can delegate this responsibility to someone who is suitably trained and has sufficient knowledge about the operation and its risks. As an FY1 doctor, you are unlikely to satisfy these criteria. Therefore, the best option is to explain your position to the registrar (C). He should then consent the patient himself or delegate the responsibility to someone else. The next best option would be to ask an appropriately qualified doctor from another team to help (D). This is not the preferred option, as such a person will have other duties, may not know the patient, and is unlikely to be part of the operating team. If ever in doubt, it is advisable to ask colleagues for advice. (E) is the first clearly wrong answer; however, it is redeemed to some extent by the fact that you are seeking advice, and an experienced nurse will probably point out that you should not consent patients for complicated procedures in FY1. The final two options—(B) and (A)—are the most unsafe. (A) is very narrowly better, as addressing the issue urgently might ensure there is time for consent taken in error to be rectified.

2. **B, E, C, A, D**

Your priority in this case must be the safety of your patient, i.e. ideally you should not perform a procedure with which you are unconfident. However, it is also important that you learn practical procedures so that you can be a full member of the team and avoid unnecessarily burdening colleagues in future. In this case, a confident fellow FY1 doctor may be the most appropriate person to assist with a relatively simple procedure. For this reason, (B) is the correct answer. As the ABG is urgent and you understand how it is performed, you should probably attempt the procedure before asking for help from a senior doctor. For this reason, (E) is the second best answer.

All doctors have varying degrees of experience and need practice to improve. Although there is no absolute requirement to inform patients how many times you have performed a procedure before, you should aim to be upfront and honest. If there is a realistic chance of failing the ABG due to inexperience, it would be polite to inform the patient first, if this would not cause them undue anxiety. For this reason, (C) is a worse option than (E).

Contacting the duty medical registrar is a less ideal option as they are likely to be dealing with unwell patients elsewhere in the hospital (A). As this is a relatively simple procedure on which you have already received training, you should think carefully before interrupting their other duties. The worst possible answer is (D) as there is no justification for handing difficult tasks over to your night colleagues; delaying the ABG risks harm to the patient, and your skills will not improve.

3. **B, D, A, C, E**

Your first priority in any patient about whom you are worried is to familiarize yourself with their details and ensure that they are stable (e.g. Airway, Breathing, Circulation). (B) is therefore the correct answer. The next best answer is (D) because hospital guidelines may ensure you manage the situation correctly and are a way of solving the problem yourself without unnecessarily overly burdening the medical registrar (A).

The two wrong answers are (C) and (E). (C) is marginally better as it is at least an attempt to identify the correct course of action. However, using unregulated online resources is commonplace but should be discouraged (C)—hospital guidelines, senior colleagues, and potentially authoritative books (e.g. *Oxford Handbook for the Foundation Programme*) are better sources of information.

The worst answer is (E) as loop diuretics are not used to manage hypernatraemia—you would have known this, had you consulted hospital guidelines or discussed with the medical registrar.

4. **A, D, C, B, E**

Doctors should understand (and be able to defend) any investigation or procedure they request. You should avoid taking responsibility for requests you do not understand, and it is particularly difficult to persuade a radiologist to accept a scan request that you do not understand yourself. Your best option is to ask the consultant (A) or, not quite as good, another member of the team (D) what the scan is for.

The other answers are incorrect. Your consultant is unlikely to appreciate you declining to request the scan (C). However, this is probably better than taking a similar approach with the radiologist (B). Although the radiologist might understand why the scan is necessary, she cannot always be expected to know what your consultant was thinking. You should aim to be better informed than this before approaching a senior doctor outside of your team.

The worst answer is clearly (E). If you have been asked to request a CT scan, you should generally not do something else simply based on your own initiative. Given that your consultant is considerably more experienced, ordering an ultrasound scan instead may both delay the definitive investigation and waste a valuable ultrasound scanning slot that could be used by someone else.

5. **B, E, D, A, C**

Thankfully, no harm came to this patient as the error was spotted by the pharmacist. The most important thing now is that both you and the organization learn from this incident.

The best answer is (B) as you must always take responsibility for your actions, although you should take steps to communicate the factors that you think contributed to the error in whatever way is necessary to effect appropriate organizational change.

(E) is the next best answer because it raises concerns about the underlying reasons for your error. It is important to take personal responsibility, but explaining your reasons to Matron in the correct way could lead to positive changes in the rota. Although (D) is a positive option, it does not raise the issue beyond your own personal reflection area and so has limited practical benefit.

(A) is not a positive option because it appears defensive and raises your concern in a forum that is unlikely to result in a constructive outcome. The worst answer is (C) because you should never seek to cover up your mistakes or ask colleagues to do so for you. If Matron feels that the error is sufficiently serious to raise with your Educational Supervisor, you should not interfere with this decision.

6. B, E, D, A, C

Patient safety is your priority and someone should follow up this test result immediately. The duty FY1 doctor is the most appropriate person to do so (B). The next best option is to visit the hospital yourself and check the test (E). Although this is of great practical inconvenience and should not be something you do frequently, it is better than the remaining options as the patient's safety can then be guaranteed.

(D) is the first wrong answer as it fails to address the immediate patient safety issue. It is, however, the best of the incorrect answers as it might stop similar problems arising in future. (A) is more incorrect as it introduces unnecessary delay and there is no guarantee that an abnormal result would have been recognized in time to treat the patient appropriately. The most incorrect answer is obviously (C).

7. A, C, B, D, E

You should first seek to clarify what has prompted your colleague's concerns. There may be good explanations or she might have noticed something that you have yet to pick up on yourself. For this reason, (A) is the best answer, and (C) would be the next most appropriate step if you acknowledged your colleague's concerns. However, it could still be an appropriate response, as you are not necessarily best placed to assess your own health and an independent assessment could be useful if others are worried. GMC guidance states that all doctors should be registered with a GP so that objective advice can be sought if necessary. You should avoid 'corridor consultations' with colleagues but could discuss this with your Educational Supervisor (B), even though they might not be qualified to assess you formally. However, it would be less appropriate to canvass the opinion of your FY1 colleagues (D). The worst answer is (E) because you should never attempt to formally assess or treat yourself.

8. C, D, E, B, A

GMC guidance states that you must always be honest and recognize the limitations of your knowledge. Your best option here is to tell the patient what you know and explain that it is the limit of your knowledge (C). (D) is the next best alternative, as it involves a suitable senior, although you may have been able to allay the patient's concerns yourself before deferring to someone else for further information. (E) suggests reflective practice and will improve your care for future patients but does not address this patient's concerns at all. Refusing to answer the patient's questions without providing a suitable alternative (e.g. speaking with a senior, finding out the answer) is even less appropriate (B). The worst answer is (A) as you do not know this for certain.

9. A, D, C, E, B

The best answer for managing acutely unwell patients always begins with 'ABCDE' and calling for help at your earliest opportunity. A patient who is clearly deteriorating quickly and whose consciousness level is falling in front of you warrants urgent assistance as you are unlikely to be able to manage a threatened airway independently on your ward. For this reason, (A) is the best answer. It is much less appropriate in the acute setting described to make a telephone call for advice when you should be busy resuscitating a patient while you are waiting for the resuscitation team to arrive (D). However, the SHO is more likely to be readily available to attend the ward and assist you than the consultant (C). (B) and (E) are the worst options only because neither recognizes that you require help in this situation. (E) is better than (B) because in the former you have at least set parameters for which you will summon help, even if you are likely to reach this point quickly given the patient's current rate of deterioration.

10. C, A, D, E, B

The key here is to strike a balance between defending yourself against an assessment that you believe is unfair and adopting a conciliatory approach so that you can learn from the perception others may have of you. To ensure a constructive meeting, you should start by asking for advice and listening to your consultant's concerns; for this reason, (C) is a better answer than (A). Part of reflecting on this experience, particularly as there is an apparent disagreement, would be to canvass the opinion of others, e.g. using the Team Assessment of Behaviour tool (D). This alone is not as good as an option as (C) and (A), which are part of the necessary dialogue with your consultant about her concerns. (B) and (E) are both incorrect; (E) is less incorrect as although your consultant is unlikely to be less than impressed about your assertion, this does not involve any other parties. The worst answer is (B) as nothing in the question indicates that there has been an irreparable breakdown in working relationships.

11. D, E, G

All doctors should be registered with a GP whom they should approach with concerns about their health (D). There is no obligation to speak with your Educational Supervisor if work is unaffected, although they may be better placed to support you if they are kept informed (E). (E) is not necessarily an incorrect answer and may be something you consider later on; however, the three correct answers listed are better. It could certainly be helpful to gain the perspective of a friend regarding your drinking habits (A). Note that in previous scenarios, wider discussions with other FY1 colleagues have been considered less ideal—in this case, the distinction has been drawn, because a friend is likely to support you and offer honest advice and be intimately aware of your drinking pattern. If your alcohol consumption has increased recently, you might wish to try reducing it for health and social reasons (G). You should not threaten your physical health by attempting to provoke withdrawal symptoms (F). You are already concerned about your drinking and should seek advice from an independent professional, rather than attempting to manage the problem further yourself (C). Although you might be concerned about acquiring an unhelpful reputation, asking your colleagues to stop gossiping (B) may be ineffective and will not solve any underlying drinking problem. Drinking secretly will certainly not resolve any such alcohol dependency (H).

12. **B, C, F**

Competence in intravenous cannulation is a fundamental skill for doctors and mandatory for successful completion of FY1.

You should identify what exactly it is you find difficult about cannulation (B), ask for supervision and feedback (C), and then seek opportunities to improve your ability (F).

Strategies to avoid cannulating patients, such as asking colleagues to do it (A), avoiding 'difficult' cases (D), or calling a specialist after a token attempt (G), will burden others and will not help you to improve your ability. Covering your own deficiencies by blaming patients (H) is not encouraged, although it might be fair to warn patients if you genuinely anticipate that multiple attempts may be necessary.

Career aspirations could be modified if you find yourself struggling (and/or not enjoying) practical procedures (E). However, it would be premature to make such decisions based on experiencing difficulties with one skill over such a short space of time.

13. **C, G, H**

GMC guidelines require all doctors to recognize the limits of their knowledge and experience. In this case, you have attempted to fluid-resuscitate the patient without success. The next step is to seek advice and/or assistance from a senior colleague (C).

As a foundation doctor, you must be able to manage patients who are potentially deteriorating until help arrives. In this case, you should ensure that there is good intravenous access (G) and that the patient is being observed carefully (H) while you are waiting for support.

Although the patient's blood pressure may be acceptable for them, this should not be assumed without further information (B). Similarly, it is far from clear that the patient is peri-arrest (D), dying (F), or appropriate for a 'Not For Resuscitation' decision (A). Inotropes would not be an appropriate next step in this case (E).

14. **A, B, E**

It is important to remain professional at all times and to take necessary steps to avoid your own feelings affecting how you behave towards others. In this case, you should recognize early on that you are behaving unprofessionally and take remedial action. It may be helpful to take a short break (A), ask a colleague for assistance (B), and address any specific factors that you think may have contributed to your behaviour (E).

Although patients should always be your priority, dealing with relatives is an important job for junior doctors, even when on call (C). Apologizing to these particular relatives (D) may well be appropriate, but the motivation for doing so should not be to avoid complaints, and it is likely that an insincere apology could inflame the situation. Clock watching is not a strong solution to the problem (H).

Action to remove relatives (F) should only be initiated if staff, patients, or other visitors are at risk. You should have sufficient insight to wonder whether two 'clashes' with relatives in quick succession may reflect your behaviour as much as theirs. The medical student (G) is not to blame!

15. **C, D, G**

You must comply as far as possible with any complaints procedure. In this case, you should cooperate with your line manager by providing factual details in a timely manner (C).

Regardless of the complaints process (and outcome), you must endeavour to improve your own practice. You may identify areas of clinical practice or communication that could be improved from this experience (D). As well as documenting carefully, you should ask for the complaint outcome (G) so as to aid the learning process.

At all times, you must be honest and trustworthy. GMC and local disciplinary procedures will expect this from all clinical staff. You must not edit the notes retrospectively to protect yourself (A) (B) or obstruct the process by not replying (E) or delaying your response (H).

Although you may need to explain your actions, being 'busy' is not an excuse for failing to examine a patient thoroughly (F). Doctors must take personal responsibility for their actions, even if other factors contribute.

16. **B, E, F**

As a junior doctor, you must recognize your own limitations at all times. In this case, you are uncomfortable with the request and must ensure patient safety, even at the expense of upsetting your consultant.

You should be honest and communicate to the consultant that you are unhappy with his request (B). It may have been miscommunicated and/or your response may prompt the consultant to change his mind. If you feel pressured to work beyond your limitations, this should be raised with your Educational Supervisor at the first available opportunity (E). If you cannot recontact the consultant, you should get in touch with another senior colleague (F) to discuss your concerns.

In this case, sedating a patient on a regular ward is likely to be unacceptable, even for a senior doctor (D). You must always prioritize patient safety over other considerations and should not comply with a request that you believe might be dangerous (A) (C) (H). Attempting to relocate the hip without sedation (G) would be very painful and may cause more harm if you are unfamiliar with the procedure.

17. **D, E, H**

You must always be open and honest about your knowledge. In this case, you should explain to the patient that you do not know the answer but will endeavour to find out (D). This will also support your development. Once you have closed any gaps in your own knowledge (H), you should carefully explain the advantages and disadvantages of CT (E). *Good Medical Practice* states that this process is a necessary part of obtaining consent for any procedure or investigation.

You should not overburden senior colleagues (C) or delay an investigation (G) if you are able to answer a question adequately after looking up the answer. This risks distracting them from their own responsibilities. You can answer any question as long as it is within your knowledge and experience to do so adequately (B).

Making up an answer (A) is dishonest unless you know it to be true. Risks, benefits, and likely consequences should be explained before a competent patient is deemed to have refused a procedure (F).

18. **A, B, H**

Wearing a watch conflicts with Department of Health policy on staff dress in clinical areas. Its removal is likely to be a reasonable request (A). You should try to accept negative feedback and use it to reflect on changes you might make in future (B). If you disagree with negative feedback, you may wish to seek other views in a genuine attempt to improve your professional appearance (H).

You may wish to raise your consultant's compliance with policy at another time (C). However, this is not an adequate defence of your own behaviour and should not be raised with another colleague in this forum. You should not provoke your registrar or act in any way that makes him feel less able to give you feedback in future (D) (E) (F).

Although bullying is an important issue for doctors, this should be distinguished from a single episode of negative feedback (G).

19. **A, B, F**

Once again, patient safety must be your first consideration. Prescribing whilst stressed, hungry, and tired is more likely to lead to errors. You must balance the risk of a prescribing error against the risk of the drug chart being delayed (F).

A single task could be done quickly before getting rest. Two drug charts may take some time and therefore you could explain your position (A) and say that you will write them later on (B).

Drug charts must sometimes be written by the on-call medical team (C) (G) as drugs cannot be given without them. However, they are a source of prescribing errors as the on-call doctor is tired, balancing multiple tasks, and may not know the patient. Prescribing should be taken seriously and not done 'quickly' before going for a break (D). Ideally, drug charts should not be written by someone who is so tired that they are nodding off to sleep (H) or who is not an authorized prescriber (E).

20. A, E, F

Doctors must be familiar with their own strengths and weaknesses. The Foundation Programme e-portfolio has a number of tools (e.g. Team Assessment of Behaviour (TAB)) for reflecting on, and so mitigating, potential weaknesses (A). Effective time management can reduce stress levels (E), as can involving senior colleagues if work levels become unmanageable (F). Although you should always aim to leave on time, this will not always be possible and doctors must be prepared to show some flexibility (D) to ensure that patients and colleagues do not come to harm.

Increasing the burden on other junior colleagues (B) (C) is unlikely to be a successful long-term strategy. Although outside interests are important, drinking excessively (G) is unhelpful and HR is unlikely to agree to time away for yoga classes. (H).

21. B, E, C, D, A

You are entitled to go home at the end of a shift. Your rota is designed to create sufficient rest so that it is within the law and guarantees patient safety. It could be convincingly argued that either (E) or (B) should be ranked first, and a fully correct answer would require you to do both of these. However, (E) implies that you are passing responsibility to the night SHO, even though he has stated that he will not accept that responsibility. It may be unfair, but to ensure patient safety that night, it may be necessary to complete urgent tasks if you have reasons to doubt that they would be completed by your colleagues (B). It is clearly correct to address the wider problem of this doctor who fails to accept this responsibility; however, in isolation, this does not address the immediate problem of tasks not being completed (C). (A) and (D) are both probably incorrect. (D) is inappropriate because there will be Trust processes that should be exhausted first, and you would always wish to take senior advice before referring a colleague to the GMC, and this should not be considered in haste when angry at 10 p.m. However, (A) must be the worst answer because it achieves nothing, except for protecting yourself with careful documentation while potentially leaving an important role within the hospital unfilled.

22. A, E, D, C, B

Doctors must sometimes work flexibly because of the unpredictable nature of their profession. However, your regular work pattern is a contractual right. Working outside these hours might conflict with the

European Working Time Directive and should potentially increase your banding supplement. This issue would be best resolved with your Clinical Supervisor, and therefore (A) is the best answer. (E) is not unreasonable; however, it is likely to result in your Educational Supervisor suggesting that you speak to your Clinical Supervisor, which takes you back to (A). (D) is the first wrong answer, although you may see this played out many times as you start work, as there are expectations in some specialties that trainees will adopt a particular approach within their specialty. It is, however, strictly wrong for the legal reasons described. (B) and (C) are clearly the worst answers. (C) is unprofessional if your consultant believes you will be working the hours he thinks that you are working. (B) has to be the worst answer because it suggests that your contracted duties during the day are neglected and it does not make it clear that anyone is taking care of your patients during this time.

23. **B, A, E, C, D**

There is a narrow margin between (A) and (B) as the correct answer. Many candidates will feel that (A) is correct as it is upfront and honest and may provoke your registrar to think of another solution. It is also likely to be the first thing you would do in this situation. When answering the SJT questions, it is important to remember that you are being asked for the most appropriate actions, and not the order of actions that you would perform. As a single intervention, it would probably be more helpful if you would take responsibility for ensuring that this task happened and then identified a way to ensure that it occurred safely. In this case, asking another suitably qualified doctor to help may be appropriate (B). There is a distinction between this sequence and a similar question (Question 1, Chapter 10, p. 73) in that here the registrar is calling from theatre and has already explained that he is unable to assist; in the other question, the registrar is on the ward and is in a much better position to consent the patient and offer guidance as to how to resolve the issue. The first wrong answer is (E) as this fails to address the clinical problem. Worse still is attempting to complete the task independently, which risks compromising the patient's safety—(C) is only marginally better than (D) as it implies there is a degree of preparation before you embark upon this unfamiliar task. Documenting your registrar's request does not absolve you of your responsibility to the patient if you perform it inappropriately and the patient comes to harm as a consequence.

24. **A, D, B, E, C**

Ideally, grave decisions of this nature should be based on a broad consensus including doctors, members of the multi-disciplinary team (MDT), relatives, and the patient herself if possible. The best answer requires you to understand the case and try to identify the reasons for your current disagreement with the family and nursing staff. It may be that an answer becomes immediately apparent, e.g. a decision to withdraw treatment has already been documented (or there may be a consensus position to be found). For this reason, (A) is the best answer. The other correct answer is to involve a senior doctor early on (D), although this will necessarily require you to understand the case before doing so, which is why it is not as good an answer as (A). The other answers are incorrect to varying degrees. (B) is probably the best because at the current time, you are responsible for directing this patient's management. If they do not have capacity (which is implied in the question), then you are obliged to make decisions in the best interests of the patient. In the absence of a more senior doctor, the arbiter of these best interests (after taking into consideration views of relatives, pre-existing wishes, etc.) could even fall to the FY1 doctor. However, it would be necessary to carefully articulate this principle and *insisting* may be the wrong approach. For the reasons stated here, (E) is worse than (B) because best interests is an objective clinical assessment and you have no discretion to delegate this responsibility to family members. Finally, the worst answer (C) is taking actions to actively hasten death, which is illegal (murder!), although inappropriate interventions can be discontinued under the doctrine of double effect.

25. **E, B, C, A, D**

Blood transfusion carries significant risks (including death) and should not be considered without good reason. The best answer is therefore (E) as there is no indication for transfusion, and this answer ensures you explain the reasons for your decision to the nurse which will hopefully ensure she is happier with the outcome. (B) is correct but not as good an answer as (E) as there is no attempt to share your reasoning with the concerned nurse. Reprimanding the nurse is probably unnecessary as she will likely be aware of the seriousness of wasting blood; you could complete the incident form, but it would probably be more appropriate if the ward team did so instead, as you have not been actively involved (C). (A) is clearly the wrong answer as it exposes the patient to the risks of an unnecessary transfusion. (D) is worst because it exposes another patient to greater harm, as you have been told in the question that the blood cannot now be returned for further use.

26. **C, D, E, B, A**

Patient safety must be your first priority. The best options are therefore (C) and (D). (C) is the better of these two because you should ensure ̲istration of the drug has not had a detrimental effect on the ̲ ̲ a close second as it would also be important to ̲ ̲ case a similar or incompatible drug was to be ̲ ̲tant only because it does not guaran- ̲ ̲ugh it goes some way towards ̲ ̲e two incorrect answers. (B) is ̲ ̲use there are nurse prescribers. ̲ ̲might see this happen on some ̲ ̲pted retrospective prescriptions. ̲ ̲scouraged at least in part because ̲ ̲re you have not verbally requested ̲ ̲tly that you asked for the drug and ̲ ̲quence. Ideally, the nurse should sign ̲ ̲ed, no prescription was signed, and a ̲ ̲cumented in the notes.

27. C, B, D, E, A

This question requires you to take some responsibility for patient welfare in an emergency, even in the presence of senior doctors, if you are not confident that they are acting correctly. You know that the correct management of a cardiac arrest begins by securing the airway. If no one else is actively managing this problem, the responsibility will fall to you (C). (B) is second best answer because, if you were not to choose managing the airway yourself, you should draw the team leader's attention to the problem in the most direct way possible. (D) is less good than (B) as it indirectly raises your concern about the airway. (E) and (A) are incorrect as both appear to ignore the threatened airway. (E) is somewhat better than (A) as you are at least offering your support.

28. E, A, C, B, D

The correct answer is (E) because a critically ill patient who is deteriorating and may be peri-arrest should be your priority, regardless of her age. (A) is less concerning because at present he is stable; however, given his presentation, you have good reason to believe he may become unstable very soon. (C) is not a lifesaving emergency, but severe pain should be accorded high priority for compassionate reasons—patients should not be left in pain when relief is available. (B) and (D) are less important because they are not *clinically* urgent. The angry relative's demand must be secondary to the immediate requirements of other patients. However, bed sores are a serious concern and you should try to discuss this situation to improve her mother's care and avert a complaint if possible. Therefore, this situation should be prioritized above the young patient awaiting discharge (D), however keen he is to go home.

29. A, B, E, C, D

The key principle at stake is that you require a patient's consent before breaching confidentiality in most circumstances. (A) is the best answer because it explains the limitations on what it is appropriate for you to do. (B) and (E) both correctly withhold the information, although (E) is less good because it is factually incorrect—there are circumstances under which you must disclose information to the police (e.g. to avert serious crime and in firearms offences).

(C) and (D) are the worst options as the outcome is passing on the d charge letter to the police against your patient's wishes. However, marginally better as this gives the patient some opportunity to r his own information.

30. B, C, E, D, A

Covering the private wing might not be one of your us ties. However, you may have a duty to help a patient in 5.0 and midway through a transfusion). For this reas answer as you would first need to assess the situatio good because you are still intending to help; ho no attempt to prioritize other routine tasks. (E) determine whether attending to tasks in the private wing is acceptable as there may be local rules.

(A) and (D) are both incorrect as you have a moral duty to help in an emergency, regardless of local arrangements or your personal feelings. Although charging the private wing for work on NHS time (D) would be improper, (A) is more incorrect as it suggests you would refuse to help, regardless of the clinical situation.

31. **A, C, E**

This patient has had an accidental overdose and needs to be reviewed as a priority (A). You must not wait until the patient shows signs of deterioration (H). Although you must not cover up clinical errors (D), the nurse may prefer to inform the Ward Sister herself (C). As this is a serious error, a formal incident report must be completed contemporaneously (E) so that a paper trail is created and lessons can be learnt. There is no need to think that this nurse is an immediate danger to other patients (B). It would be inappropriate to discuss with intensive care (F) until you have assessed the patient and have decided that higher-level care is necessary. Intravenous fluids and vomiting are not standard interventions (G) and would only be indicated on senior advice or if directed by a reliable resource (e.g. Toxbase®).

32. **A, D, F**

You should be sensitive to the daughter's concern but firm that you cannot breach confidentiality in this case (A). You may indicate that you have not been given permission to give details to anyone (D). It might be helpful to let your patient know that close family members are anxious for details (F) in case she changes her mind and agrees to involve them. Calling security (B) is an overreaction and likely to inflame the situation. You must not lie (C) or breach your patient's confidentiality (E), even if you feel coerced by her family. Capacity is not age-dependent (G) and cannot be assumed to be lacking in an elderly patient. Your consultant is unlikely to approve of his contact details being given out (H)—colleagues are also entitled to a degree of confidentiality.

33. **B, C, D**

You have a duty to speak out whenever you feel that patient care is being compromised. In this case, you should let a senior know (B) if you are unable to cope—they might be able to help or redirect resources accordingly. A clear jobs list will help you prioritize tasks so that the most urgent are completed first (C). You must not neglect potentially unwell patients to meet other commitments (e.g. hospital targets) (D), even if you document the reason (E). However, you should not be discourteous or facetious when declining to help the Emergency Department (H), in order to maintain good working relations. Time spent on a coffee break (F) or drafting a letter (G) could be better used to assess your potentially unwell patients. You should never render yourself uncontactable (A) in case emergencies require your immediate attention.

34. A, C, H

If the CT request is very urgent, you should alert your consultant (A) if there is any reason why it cannot go ahead. You might have miscommunicated its urgency and/or he might want to intervene. You should take some time to compose yourself and speak to a supportive colleague if one is available (C). If you are finding things particularly difficult, you should seek independent advice from your GP, Educational Supervisor, and/or Occupational Health (H). Talking again to the radiologist (D) or asking a colleague to do so (G) is unlikely to be helpful unless the situation has changed or more facts are available.

The radiologist may have good reason to decline your request and is not necessarily being obstructive (E). In any event, the Medical Director would not be your first port of call. You should only ask to go home (F) if you cannot continue working, as this may disrupt patient care and is unlikely to resolve your difficulties. A generic email asking others to shoulder your work (B) might be misinterpreted and/or unfairly burden colleagues.

35. B, E, G

You should not accept a situation that compromises patient care and your first action should be to reason with the SHO (B). This should be done in a non-confrontational manner; however, speaking directly to the SHO (A) is likely to result in a swifter resolution or compromise than involving the consultant (E). You should let nursing colleagues know in advance that you might be slower to respond than usual (G). However, you should never discourage staff from calling you about deteriorating patients (C)—more can be done for unwell patients who are identified early.

If the ward team is short-staffed, you should not seek to leave your SHO alone to cope (D). The SHO might be a surgical trainee who will learn more (and be more useful) in theatre than an FY1 doctor. You must not fake illness (F) as this is dishonest and unfair to colleagues who will be even more stretched the following day. Patient discharges should not be delayed unnecessarily (H) but might be lower priority than some tasks.

36. B, C, E

FY1 doctors must remain resilient under pressure. In this case, you should try to ignore the camera (B) and act normally by explaining politely that you cannot discuss a patient's case without their permission (C). Do not breach confidentiality simply because the situation is pressurized (F). You have a right not to feel threatened at work and should call security for assistance if you feel out of your depth (E). Trying to obscure (A) or confiscate (H) the camera will aggravate the situation and look very bad on tape afterwards! You should not lie under any circumstances (G) but politely decline to answer questions. Although directing relatives to the correct member of staff (D) might be helpful, the result in this case would simply be to shift an uncomfortable situation onto a nursing colleague.

37. **A, E, H**

There are very few circumstances that justify dishonesty and this is not one of them. You should not complete the questionnaires with false data (A) (B). However, you should recognize your omission and let your senior doctor know your plan to improve the following week (E). Empathizing with the senior doctor and demonstrating that you understand their importance (H) will help defuse any potential conflict. Refusing outright to participate (F) is likely to result in conflict and is at odds with your status as a Trust employee. However, the questionnaires need to be prioritized, alongside other tasks, and an afternoon calling patients for this purpose is poor use of clinical time (G). Lying to a senior doctor, even if this might appear to solve the problem, is unjustifiable and could result in professional difficulties (D). Raising concerns with a newspaper in the first instance would be likely to result in employment and/or professional disciplinary action (C).

38. **C, A, H**

You cannot prevent a patient with capacity from leaving hospital and the patient should be aware that he is free to leave at any time (C) (B). However, you have a duty to ensure that he understands the associated risks and you should find these out if you are unsure (A) (F). If you are concerned about the patient's decision, you might consult a senior doctor (H) who could potentially counsel the patient more convincingly. It is clearly wrong to place the burden of looking up risks on to the patient (F).

If your consultant has made a clinical plan, you should not contradict this without very good reason (D) (E). FY1 doctors must be open to patients having different values and life priorities. It is acceptable for a patient to prioritize a family engagement (G) as long as he understands the potential consequences of doing so.

39. **C, F, H**

Although, ideally, you should not work when exhausted, it would be more dangerous for you to leave without a replacement (D) or to become uncontactable (B). You should continue working (F) but let a manager know at the earliest opportunity so that relief can be sought (C) (E). As you are due to work the following night, the manager should arrange sufficient cover so that you are not still exhausted on returning to the hospital (H). You must continue to review patients who are potentially unwell, even if you are tired (G).

Your FY1 colleague should not come to work with diarrhoea and vomiting as there is a risk of spreading norovirus to vulnerable patients (A).

40. **A, C, E**

Although the patient has dementia, you should first try to communicate with him as with any patient (A). As he has already hit a healthcare assistant, he may continue to be violent and need to be restrained. Security officers are the most appropriate people for this task (C). Once the situation is controlled, you should attend to any injuries arising, including to staff (E). You should not do anything likely to scare the patient (F) or cause harm (B) and should treat him with as much dignity as the situation permits. An AMTS assessment is unlikely to be successful or add very much to his immediate management (D). FY1 doctors should not give anaesthetic drugs (G), let alone in an unmonitored ward environment— propofol is not a solution in this case.

An agitated patient risks harming themselves or others and therefore is the responsibility of all staff (H).

41. C, E, D, B, A

You should respect the fact that your colleague likely has other pressing responsibilities while also ensuring the safety of your own patient. If you have not been able to contact the medical registrar about a deteriorating patient, the best answer is to escalate further and obtain senior support from your own consultant (C). It should go without saying that you would continue adjusting your management according to new findings as best as you can (E). You are unlikely to achieve much more by paging again (B) and additional delay may be harmful (D). (A) is the worst option as it does not help the patient who is immediately at risk and ignores the likely explanation that the medical registrar might well be unable to move away from a patient that is sicker than the one for which you are currently responsible.

42. B, A, E, C, D

It is important to accommodate reasonable requests if this will make patients more comfortable and assist with delivering effective care. This has to be balanced against ensuring that unreasonable demands do not deprive other patients of resources. The polite and simple response would be to enquire what the concerns were (B) as they may be easy to understand and address. For example, the request might conceal that the patient wants a female doctor because she may need a pelvic examination. If there happened to be a female Muslim doctor working with you in A&E, you may both decide to accommodate the request (A), although this should not usually be to the detriment of other patients. You could involve your consultant, but it would be unlikely to result in any alternative action (E). Involving the hospital imam would be unnecessary and delay addressing the underlying problem (C). Option (D) is clearly unfair and potentially unsafe.

43. A, C, E

You need to be pragmatic in organizing scheduled meetings with supervisors, but they should occur within reasonable time frame. The best options are those in which you are proactive. Options (A), (B), and (C) are sensible strategies for trying to accommodate this meeting or looking for an alternative suggestion via your supervisor. The other options are unhelpful and impractical in trying to resolve the problem

(F) (H) or escalate the issue prematurely (D) (E). Option (G) does not meet your educational needs and would be dishonest.

44. **A, D, H**

It is clear that the patient has anxieties that need to be addressed (A) and the scenario does not suggest evidence of an underlying sinister cause (H). It would be reasonable to ask a more senior colleague, both to ensure you have not missed anything and to help further reassure the patient (D). It is rarely proper to request investigations or referrals that are not indicated, even if the patient is very concerned (B) (E). His anxiety does not appear to warrant medication or inpatient treatment by itself, given the facts in the stem (F) (G). It would be dishonest to pretend to examine the patient again (C).

45. **A, E, B, D, C**

Emergency departments will likely have their own policies regarding how they deal with these requests, which can occur fairly frequently. Whatever the policy, the nurse in charge would be the best person to consult in the first instance (A). Otherwise, a sensible strategy would be to politely refuse the request as it is not a sustainable strategy to pay the taxi fare for every patient that asks (E). Paying out of your own pocket might seem kind but might be misconstrued and certainly risks building expectations that other healthcare professionals might do the same (B). It is not clear that the vulnerable adult protection team has a role to play (D), but the worst option is (C), which suggests being complicit in misuse of hospital resources.

Chapter 11

Effective communication

Introduction

Communication is fundamental to the role of the doctor. It includes routine verbal communication (e.g. history taking, updating relatives, handovers, and requesting investigations from specialists), written communication (e.g. prescriptions, updating the clinical notes, and discharge summaries), breaking bad news, and 'challenging' interactions such as dealing with an angry relative.

Questions within this section assess your ability to communicate effectively with patients and colleagues. Effective communication requires understanding and being understood.

You will need to demonstrate an ability to negotiate with colleagues, to document information within the medical notes clearly and concisely, to gather information from patients, and to listen to angry relatives. As always, your responses must adapt to the needs and context of each situation, while always remembering to demonstrate empathy and compassion.

- Listen to patients, relatives, and colleagues. They are trying to tell you something.
- Explain your position carefully after listening to the other side.
- Adapt your style as far as possible to the person with whom you are communicating.
- However strongly you feel, poor manners will never get the job done faster.

Foundation doctors should not usually be left to 'break bad news' in the classical sense of a new cancer diagnosis in clinic. However, bad news can take many forms and it is likely that you will find yourself going through the 'breaking bad news' sequence many times during the foundation programme. For example, the following scenarios are all bad news to varying degrees. Some patients will take such developments in their stride and others will rank them amongst other significant life events.

- An incidental 'nodule' found on a CT chest that might be benign but will require a follow-up scan in three months.
- An elderly man who has become very unwell and is unlikely to survive while you are on call. You have been assigned the task of calling his wife, providing an update, and suggesting she come to the hospital urgently.
- The fact that investigations have all been normal and they are being discharged without a diagnosis for their persistent debilitating abdominal pain. This might be as disappointing for some patients as a new diagnosis or the possibility of a lurking cancer.

The Foundation Programme Curriculum is explicit that FY1 doctors should be able to demonstrate that they 'break bad news compassionately and supportively'.

Fortunately, although the textbook 'angry relative' comes up frequently in communication skills OSCE stations, they are encountered much less often in real life. However, like breaking bad news, you might well have to implement the 'angry relative' principles on a regular basis when you find yourself communicating with people that are disappointed, disgruntled, scared, and/or frustrated. In general, the following principles apply:

- Remain calm and avoid getting angry in response.
- Listen actively by keeping eye contact and nodding to acknowledge their words where appropriate.
- Ask open questions and try to find out more about what has happened and why they are upset.
- Acknowledge deficiencies in care and apologize when it is appropriate to do so.

References and further reading

UK Foundation Programme Office (2016). *The Foundation Programme Curriculum 2016*. http://www.foundationprogramme.nhs.uk/curriculum/

QUESTIONS

1. You are covering medical wards at the weekend when you are asked by a nurse to speak to the relatives of a patient about his newly diagnosed malignancy. You have not met the patient before but are told that his relatives are very anxious.

Rank in order the following actions in response to this situation (1 = Most appropriate; 5 = Least appropriate)

A Establish how much the relatives wish to know, and respond to their requests honestly and with compassion.

B Politely decline to discuss the health of the patient without his explicit permission.

C Ask the nurse to read the medical notes and speak to the family after doing so.

D Explain that you do not know the patient and that they should speak to the regular ward team instead.

E Collectively address both the patient's and the family's concerns, and answer each of their questions in turn.

2. You are a respiratory FY1 doctor and have inserted a number of chest drains before and have been asked to do so for a patient on your ward. Previous consents have always been obtained by different doctors. You intend to obtain consent for this patient but recall that this can be found to be invalid afterwards unless the patient is warned about important complications.

Rank in order the following actions in response to this situation (1 = Most appropriate; 5 = Least appropriate)

A Obtain verbal consent, and document that the patient has been consented in the notes.

B Obtain legal advice before consenting.

C Obtain verbal consent, with a nurse as a witness.

D Complete a formal written consent form.

E Refuse to complete the procedure as only SHO grade or above should consent.

3. You are working as an FY1 doctor at night in the surgical assessment unit, when you are asked to clerk an elderly patient who is profoundly deaf and unable to write.

Rank in order the following actions in response to this situation (1 = Most appropriate; 5 = Least appropriate)

A Attempt a brief verbal history.

B Skip the history, and focus your management on the examination and investigations.

C Do not attempt to clerk the patient without an interpreter present.

D Complete your detailed history via handwritten questions.

E Extrapolate a history, based on the limited findings of the ambulance crew on their initial assessment sheet.

4. Your next patient at the gynaecology clinic arrives with her brother-in-law, who explains that she is unable to speak any English. As you begin the interview, you start to suspect that her brother-in-law is only communicating some of the information.

Rank in order the following actions in response to this situation (1 = Most appropriate; 5 = Least appropriate)

A Reiterate to the brother-in-law that you need him to translate word for word.

B Try to establish whether the patient is happy with her brother-in-law acting as interpreter.

C Schedule another appointment with a formal interpreter.

D Invite the clinic receptionist into the consultation, as she claims to speak a similar language to the patient's.

E Ask the brother-in-law to leave and complete the consultation without any interpreter.

5. You are on a busy orthopaedic ward round with your consultant when a nurse mentions that one of your patients drinks 60 units of alcohol per week. He is scheduled for an elective knee replacement in two days but is otherwise fit and healthy.

Choose the THREE most appropriate actions to take in this situation

A Ask the consultant to review the issue during the ward round.

B Return to the patient after the ward round to discuss the matter further with him.

C Prescribe Pabrinex® and chlordiazepoxide while the consultant consents the patient.

D Discuss the matter further with the patient during the ward round.

E Tell the patient to stop drinking alcohol.

F Mention the issue to the registrar after the ward round.

G Ask the nurse to keep superfluous information until after the ward round to avoid interruptions.

H Inform the drug and alcohol services representative.

6. A 50-year-old is admitted to hospital with a severe sudden-onset headache, which you think is probably a migraine. Your registrar asks you to telephone the on-call radiologist at home to authorize an urgent CT scan. You become distracted completing other jobs for the registrar and only remember to telephone the radiologist an hour later.

Rank in order the following actions in response to this situation (1 = Most appropriate; 5 = Least appropriate)

A Inform the registrar about the delay and phone the radiologist immediately to request the CT head scan.

B Phone the radiologist and explain that the registrar only just asked you to arrange the CT scan.

C Phone the radiologist and explain that the registrar wants the CT head scan, but you think that it is likely to be a migraine.

D Ask the registrar to call the consultant radiologist himself.

E Phone your own consultant and ask for advice first.

7. At the end of your shift, you are told that a new patient has arrived under the care of your team. The nurse reads a long list of jobs that need completing and asks if you would address these before leaving. This is the third consecutive day that you will leave the ward late.

Rank in order the following actions in response to this situation (1 = Most appropriate; 5 = Least appropriate)

A Leave and review the jobs in the morning.

B Review the jobs and perform those that will take less than 15 minutes.

C Review the jobs that appear most urgent and complete these before handing over to the on-call doctor.

D Ask the nurses to contact the on-call doctor who can then review the patient.

E Ask the nurses to do what they can and to contact the on-call doctor if they feel that anything else must be done before the next morning.

8. You are the surgical FY1 doctor on call and are assessing an acutely unwell patient. This takes you until the end of your shift and leads to the accumulation of many ward jobs. The overnight surgical FY2 doctor to whom you hand over is infuriated with your 'slow pace' and threatens to complain to your consultant in the morning unless you assist her.

Choose the THREE most appropriate actions to take in this situation

A Apologize for your failure to complete the ward jobs.

B Ask for feedback in order to improve your management and handover.

C Offer to continue working up the previously unwell patient who is now stabilized.

D Offer to assist with the ward jobs until she feels that the list of jobs has become more manageable.

E Do not hand her any more jobs, in an effort to avoid antagonizing her.

F Explain that you are unable to complete any more jobs, now that your shift is over.

G Phone the surgical registrar in order to help resolve the apparent conflict.

H Complain to her consultant in the morning.

9. You are an FY1 doctor in rheumatology, looking after a patient who is about to be discharged this afternoon. During his stay, a computed tomography pulmonary angiography (CTPA) was completed for chest pain which was negative but showed a lung mass of unknown significance, with a suggestion for interval scanning.

Rank in order the following actions in response to this situation (1 = Most appropriate; 5 = Least appropriate)

A Use capital letters in the discharge letter to highlight the incidental finding and requirement for an interval CT scan.

B Phone the GP to inform them of this finding.

C Explain the problem to the patient and ensure he sees his GP to arrange an interval CT scan.

D Inform the ward clerk to relay the report findings to the patient.

E Advise that the patient returns to the rheumatology clinic to see your consultant for further review of the mass.

10. As the FY1 doctor for a medical team, you are seeing a patient for the first time on the Monday ward round. You realize that the admitting doctors on Friday did not arrange a review by the weekend medical team, despite grossly abnormal blood results. What would you include as part of your written entry in the medical notes?

Choose the THREE most appropriate in this situation

A Your opinion as to whether it was appropriate to be reviewed by the weekend medical team.

B 'This patient was not seen by a weekend review team.'

C Medical entries for the weekend by assessing the patient retrospectively.

D Both Friday's and Monday's blood results.

E Today's blood results only.

F Today's management plan.

G Avoid writing anything, but review the patient.

H Tell the patient that the doctors treating him initially had done so incorrectly.

11. Your consultant asks you to insert a peripheral cannula into the vein of a large 14-year-old boy with learning difficulties. His parents are very anxious about the procedure, after the distress caused during previous attempts at venepuncture. They ask whether a sedative could be used just before the procedure.

Choose the THREE most appropriate actions to take in this situation

A Trick the boy into having the cannula inserted by hiding the equipment from him until the last possible moment.

B Use a play therapist to familiarize the patient with the procedure, even though this might take several hours.

C Explain to the parents that you will insert the cannula in the middle of the night when the patient is least likely to resist.

D Explain to the parents that it would be safer to physically restrain the child.

E Explore the anxieties of the parents before pursuing a mutually agreed plan.

F Offer to use an intramuscular sedative to 'help him sleep' during the procedure.

G Ask to cannulate the parents first in order to demonstrate the procedure to the patient.

H Talk to the patient to see how he would feel about the procedure.

12. You are involved in a clinical research project, taking consent for the collection of an additional oesophageal biopsy during oesophagogastroduodenoscopy (OGD). A patient with long-standing gastric reflux disease arrives for her regular OGD. She is very pleasant and accommodating but is known to be anxious prior to OGD procedures.

Rank in order the following actions in response to this situation (1 = Most appropriate; 5 = Least appropriate)

A As she is anxious and unlikely to want further information, briefly explain that she can help with medical research if she signs a consent form.

B Explain the complications from the OGD and how one additional biopsy adds very little to her total risk from the procedure.

C Try to alleviate her future anxiety by explaining that she is participating in a trial that will eventually lead to the development of less invasive methods of oesophageal examination.

D Take the extra biopsy, but wait until after the procedure to obtain consent from the patient and before using any of the samples for research.

E Do not include the patient in the study, given her level of anxiety.

13. You are looking after several unwell patients as the medical FY1 doctor covering wards at the weekend, when a Ward Sister asks you for an urgent discharge summary to help relieve a bed crisis in the hospital. She sympathizes with your workload but insists that a discharge letter must be written immediately.

Rank in order the following actions in response to this situation (1 = Most appropriate; 5 = Least appropriate)

A Acknowledge the severity of the bed crisis, but refer her to your registrar, explaining that you have more urgent matters to attend to.

B Phone the registrar and ask if there are any spare junior doctors who can assist with your tasks.

C Offer to write the discharge letter once you have stabilized your patients.

D Ask the Ward Sister to complete the discharge letter but sign a blank copy in advance to expedite the discharge.

E Take two minutes to write a brief discharge letter before returning to the care of your patients.

14. A patient with newly diagnosed terminal lung cancer asks to see you on the general medicine ward. He would like to make a complaint about your registrar, whom he feels has failed to offer him treatment that might prolong his life.

Rank in order the following actions in response to this situation (1 = Most appropriate; 5 = Least appropriate)

A Empathize with the patient's traumatic experience and offer to raise the matter with the registrar and consultant.

B Defend the registrar's actions, highlighting their knowledge and experience, and the generally poor prognosis of most lung cancers irrespective of the treatment modality.

C Explore the patient's concerns further.

D Inform the patient that you will refer him to the oncologist to consider chemo-/radiotherapy.

E Offer him the services of an appropriate religious leader to address any spiritual questions he may have.

15. You are working in a team of three surgical FY1 doctors. Tim, one of the surgical FY1 doctors, leaves the ward on time every day but routinely fails to complete his daily tasks. You decide to address the matter after leaving another shift more than an hour late in order to complete Tim's tasks.

Rank in order the following actions in response to this situation (1 = Most appropriate; 5 = Least appropriate)

A Share any additional workload between yourself and the other surgical FY1 doctor, without involving Tim in the matter.

B Inform Tim of your additional workload and ask him whether he is experiencing any difficulties in completing his routine jobs.

C Speak to your other surgical FY1 colleague and encourage her not to complete Tim's routine tasks.

D Demand that Tim arranges a meeting with his Foundation and Clinical Supervisors in order to 'address his failings'.

E Inform your consultant.

16. Phlebotomy rounds have been cancelled. You delegate venesection to your ward team. A nurse refuses to take blood from a patient who is being investigated for human immunodeficiency virus (HIV).

Rank in order the following actions in response to this situation (1 = Most appropriate; 5 = Least appropriate)

A Explain the ethical responsibility of medical staff to all patients.

B Demand that the nurse attempts to take the blood sample, or else she will be reported.

C Ask about her concerns about the task and what could be done to improve her confidence in this situation.

D Take the sample yourself.

E Instruct another nurse to take the sample, but avoid telling them about the patient's possible HIV status to avoid frightening them.

17. You are preparing to finish your ward shift and must leave on time to catch a flight to the test centre where you are due to sit an important examination. There are still two patients left to see as part of your ward round. Both are stable and awaiting input from social services, but your visit is likely to be prolonged by family members who are currently visiting.

Rank in order the following actions in response to this situation (1 = Most appropriate; 5 = Least appropriate)

A Perform a quick examination of each patient without speaking to them or their families.

B See the patients, but explain that you cannot spend much time with their relatives today and that someone will be available to answer questions tomorrow.

C Ask the nurses to remove the families before briefly reviewing each patient.

D Assess the patients as usual and answer any questions the family members may have, even if this results in missing your flight.

E Explain to the nurses that the patients will be seen on tomorrow's ward round, and catch your flight.

18. You are interested in orthopaedic surgery and have been asked to 'scrub in' and assist with a total knee replacement. The orthopaedic surgeon is willing to spend longer with you in theatre, provided that you consent the patient. You have not obtained consent for a surgical procedure before, but understand about some possible complications.

Rank in order the following actions in response to this situation (1 = Most appropriate; 5 = Least appropriate)

A Admit to the patient that you are unfamiliar with consenting for the procedure but that he can ask the consultant later on if he has questions that you cannot answer.

B Attempt to consent the patient, and refer any specific questions to the anaesthetist who will conduct a preoperative assessment later on.

C Refuse to consent the patient.

D Ask the consultant to run through the procedure with you before consenting the patient.

E Ask the surgical registrar to consent the patient.

19. You are asked to speak to a new patient who is a suspected intravenous drug user and has been admitted recently following an opiate overdose. He has repeatedly been asked to stay in bed but continues to wander and demands to be allowed to leave.

Rank in order the following actions in response to this situation (1 = Most appropriate; 5 = Least appropriate)

A Explain the nature of his admission and the dangers of discharge, and reiterate the risk of death if he were to self-discharge.

B Explore his reasons for wanting to self-discharge.

C Obtain the details of his family and ask them to get involved.

D Address any concerns or approaches adopted by the nursing staff that may be antagonizing the patient.

E Do not attempt to engage with a person who has recently used intra-venous drugs, as they are unlikely to be cooperative.

20. You have been asked to complete a death certificate for a patient whose care you were briefly involved in during the last few days of his life. There were no suspicious circumstances surrounding his death, but you are unclear about its precise cause. The mortuary staff suggest that you speak with someone else first if you are not sure.

Choose the THREE most appropriate actions to take in this situation

A Telephone your consultant.

B Telephone your registrar.

C Telephone the duty pathologist.

D Telephone the coroner's officer.

E Contact the ward clerk.

F Contact the nursing staff who looked after the patient.

G Telephone the patient's next of kin.

H Telephone the local police.

21. You are clerking a young child in accident and emergency (A&E) who has been admitted with suspected bronchiolitis. Physical examination is unremarkable, except for a moderate wheeze, although you note that the parents appear somewhat unkempt, with dirty hands and clothes. You consider what to document as part of your findings in the medical notes.

Rank in order the following in response to this situation (1 = Most appropriate; 5 = Least appropriate)

A Your opinion of the parents' treatment of the child, based on their appearance.

B Detailed physical examination and objective clinical assessment of the child.

C A brief summary of your clinical assessment.

D Complete your notes after they have been confirmed by a senior.

E Complete your notes later on after getting through a few more patients, to keep the clinic moving.

22. You are working as the only junior doctor for the orthogeriatric team, assessing a patient who has had a fall. You are bleeped by a nurse on another ward about one of your outliers who has become febrile. While you are taking this call, your crash bleep starts to sound.

Rank in order the following actions in response to this situation (1 = Most appropriate; 5 = Least appropriate)

A Document your current assessment of the patient who has fallen and then attend to your other commitments.

B Attend the crash call and then return to write in the notes retrospectively for the fallen patient.

C Attend the crash call and then see the pyrexial patient before documenting your assessment of the patient who fell.

D Avoid documenting the fallen patient as you are likely to be distracted by other tasks after attending the crash call and seeing the pyrexial patient.

E Allow other members of the crash team to attend the arrest while you complete all your documentation.

23. You are working alone in the afternoon on your colorectal ward as the FY1 doctor being shadowed by a final-year medical student. The nurse informs you that a patient is looking increasingly unwell, a peripheral venous cannula needs siting for a blood transfusion, and another patient's family wishes to speak with you in private.

Choose the THREE most appropriate actions to take in this situation

A Assess the unwell patient alone.

B Assess the unwell patient with the medical student.

C Ask the medical student to assess the patient alone, and join him as soon as possible.

D Ask the student whether he wishes to try to place the peripheral venous cannula.

E Attempt to insert the peripheral venous cannula yourself.

F Speak to the patient's family with a nurse present.

G Speak alone to the patient's family.

H Ask the student whether he would be comfortable speaking to the family.

24. While you are working in A&E, a nurse informs you that a 33-week pregnant woman is being brought by helicopter into resuscitation, following a road traffic collision. She asks you to prepare for her arrival in approximately five minutes. Your registrar has already been informed, and he asks you to call for assistance while he bleeps the obstetric team.

Choose the THREE most appropriate actions to take in this situation

A Inform the neonatal registrar.

B Call the orthopaedic consultant at home.

C Fast bleep the haematology registrar.

D Summon the cardiac arrest team.

E Request phototherapy light.

F Call the switchboard and ask them to put out a trauma call.

G Ask a nurse to find a neonatal incubator and bring it to resuscitation.

H Ensure that there are medical students present, to maximize the learning opportunity.

25. While working on call, you are asked to cannulate a large patient who requires intravenous antibiotics for a suspected diarrhoeal infection. Your bleep sounds for a third time during your fourth cannulation attempt when you finally believe that you have obtained access.

Rank in order the following actions in response to this situation (1 = Most appropriate; 5 = Least appropriate)

A Stop your attempt immediately and answer your bleep.

B Secure and flush the cannula before answering your bleep.

C Try to get the attention of the Ward Sister so that she can answer your bleep.

D Answer your bleep after securing and flushing the cannula, cleaning the work area, and saying goodbye to the patient.

E Ignore the bleep as they will call again if it is important.

26. A patient on your ward is diagnosed with anal cancer. He tells you that his community would react very negatively if they knew of his diagnosis. As a result, he is very anxious that no one finds out, including his family.

Rank in order the following actions in response to this situation (1 = Most appropriate; 5 = Least appropriate)

A Promise to remove any mention of anal cancer from his notes.

B Tell the patient that you will remove any mention of his diagnosis from patient lists.

C Tell the patient that his family are bound to find out at some point and it would be better if he told them.

D Let the nursing staff know that his family are not aware of the diagnosis.

E Treat him as any other patient under your care.

27. You hear Karen, one of the nurses, speaking unpleasantly to a child on the paediatric ward. The child is known to be particularly challenging to work with and has a history of learning difficulties and behavioural problems.

Rank in order the following actions in response to this situation (1 = Most appropriate; 5 = Least appropriate)

A Approach the pair, and ask to speak to Karen.

B Speak to a senior nurse before approaching Karen.

C Ask other staff working on the ward whether they have noticed any inappropriate behaviour recently.

D Do not raise any concerns as the child is not at risk.

E Inform the hospital Trust.

36. The palliative care nurse asks you to join her for a meeting with Jenny, whose husband is close to the end of life. You have been on leave for the last two weeks and are not familiar with the patient. Your seniors are all in clinic and you are alone on the ward.

Rank in order the following actions in response to this situation (1 = Most appropriate; 5 = Least appropriate)

A Agree to see Jenny with the nurse, after reading through the medical notes.

B Ask the nurse to familiarize you with the case details before meeting Jenny.

C Agree to be present during any discussion but not to answer any medical questions.

D Ask the palliative care nurse if she can wait until your seniors are back from clinic as they know the patient better.

E Go into the meeting and pick up the story as the nurse talks to Jenny.

37. The registrar asks you to book a foot X-ray for a patient on the orthopaedic ward. When booking the scan, you are only able to find an option for 'CT foot'. He asks you to book a CT scan but call radiology to amend the request. You are apprehensive about this strategy as you have previously seen it lead to inappropriate imaging.

Rank in order the following actions in response to this situation (1 = Most appropriate; 5 = Least appropriate)

A Book a CT foot scan and then call radiology to amend your request.

B Voice your concerns and explain that you have seen this strategy fail before.

C Speak with radiology first, and then book the 'CT foot'.

D Complete a clinical incident form about the registrar's willingness to compromise patient safety.

E Ask the registrar to book the scan under his name.

38. Your consultant is about to close the abdomen after a very long emergency laparotomy. He is a formidable personality and earlier told you to stop talking so that he could concentrate on finishing the operation. Although you have not been paying full attention, you think that a swab might have been left behind but are far from certain.

Rank in order the following actions in response to this situation (1 = Most appropriate; 5 = Least appropriate)

A Immediately inform the consultant of your suspicion.

B Ask the scrub nurse to recount the swabs.

C Ask another question to 'break the ice', before raising the possibility of a swab being left in the abdomen.

D Remain quiet as you were not really paying attention.

E Ask an indirect question such as: 'How harmful would it be if a swab was left in the abdominal cavity?'

39. Your consultant has agreed to complete a work-based assessment for you on numerous occasions but has not yet done so. The deadline for completion of all assessments is approaching.

Rank in order the following actions in response to this situation (1 = Most appropriate; 5 = Least appropriate)

A Ask for your consultant's login details to complete the form yourself.

B Find another consultant to complete a work-based assessment.

C Let the foundation school know that you are having difficulty finding assessors.

D Remind your consultant that the deadline is approaching.

E Let your Educational Supervisor know you are having difficulty finding assessors.

40. You have clerked Mr Smith, a 56-year-old man with abdominal pain, who was also reviewed by Dr Mayer, the duty consultant. The following day, the new duty consultant reads your clerking and proposes a completely different management plan. He has no new information to hand and did not examine the patient, and you are unhappy with his suggestions.

Rank in order the following actions in response to this situation (1 = Most appropriate; 5 = Least appropriate)

A Politely decline to follow the second consultant's management plan until he sees the patient.

B Clarify with the second consultant to whom you are ultimately responsible.

C Highlight the differences in management between the two consultants.

D Accept the plan instigated by the second consultant.

E Ask the registrar to see the patient afterwards for a 'tie-breaker' opinion.

41. Another FY1 complains to you that they are not receiving any teaching during their haematology placement. This problem had been raised by another colleague, although you are revising for a forthcoming surgical exam.

Choose the THREE most appropriate actions to take in this situation

A Acknowledge your colleague's concerns, but explain you would prefer not to receive teaching as you are busy with your own revision.

B Volunteer to offer surgical teaching to your colleague

C Approach a registrar in the team who might be interested in offering teaching

D Suggest to the department head to organize a week of teaching.

E Get together as a group of FY1s and ask the consultants whether they could incorporate teaching into the daily ward round

F Suggest that your FY1 colleague begins revision for their own intended specialty exam.

G Record this feedback on the 'end of placement' survey.

H Inform the Medical Director

42. You read on a non-medical friend's social media page that a consultant in your hospital was rude to her while she was a patient. Your friend appears very upset and is thinking about writing a complaint.

Choose the THREE most appropriate actions to take in this situation

A Contact your friend privately for further details about what happened.

B Inform the consultant responsible of the allegations and assess his response before determining whether to pursue the matter further.

C Provide her with advice about the hospital complaints system, including PALS.

D Ask your medical defence organization.

E Forward your friend's page to the hospital's media team.

F Ignore the issue; unless a formal complaint is made, it is not your responsibility.

G Suggest that the friend should not challenge the behaviour until she has completed her treatment at the hospital.

H Re-arrange your friend's future appointments to avoid encountering the same consultant.

43. Three teams are involved with specialist input for a long-term patient on your elderly care ward with dementia. The patients' wife complains they are confused about conflicting management plans from all the doctors, which is making her husband very distressed.

Rank in order the following actions in response to this situation (1 = Most appropriate; 5 = Least appropriate)

A Establish what is currently understood.

B Arrange a meeting with consultants from all three teams.

C Ask your elderly care registrar to join you.

D Spend some time reviewing the medical notes to familiarize yourself with the various plans.

E Explain that you are busy with other patients but that PALS might be able to help.

44. You overhear a locum consultant explaining a procedure to a patient. You feel the consultant's explanation is unclear and worry about his difficulty communicating with patients, since English is his second language.

Choose the THREE most appropriate actions to take in this situation

A Assess whether harming patient safety.

B Check whether achieved his professional qualifications.

C Inform the immigration authority.

D Speak with your Educational Supervisor.

E Ask the patient afterwards whether he has any questions about the procedure.

F Speak with the ward nurse to see if they have any concerns.

G Approach the consultant's secretary.

H Speak with the consultant about your concerns.

45. You are an FY1 on the respiratory ward and have been managing a patient with COPD, who is due for discharge after staying on the ward for 2 months. He is reluctant to go home and is becoming angry and upset.

Rank in order the following actions in response to this situation (1 = Most appropriate; 5 = Least appropriate)

A Speak to the patient's family, to try to convince him to leave.

B Accept the patient's wishes.

C Complete his discharge paperwork, regardless of the patient's reluctance to stay.

D Explain that he is safe to be discharged, there are risks of being in hospital, and the bed is needed for other patients.

E Call security.

ANSWERS

1. **B, E, D, C, A**

(B) is the only correct answer, as you do not know the patient, the relationship with their family, and what each party already knows about the condition. In most circumstances, it is necessary to gain express consent before discussing with relatives, and this becomes even more important in the context of a serious discussion, e.g. a new diagnosis of cancer. Therefore, (A) is the worst answer as it implies that you have not sought consent from the patient, despite subsequent steps being correct. By talking to the family in the presence of the patient, you are giving the patient an opportunity to indicate they are unhappy about further information being disclosed, and they are present when any information is shared. Therefore, (E) is the next best answer. Although usually it would be more appropriate for the day team to deal with this, as they know the case much better and can provide continuity, we are told the family is anxious and it would be inhumane to leave them uninformed if the patient agreed to a discussion at this time; hence, (D) is less appropriate than (E). (C) is a bad option, as this is not the nurse's primary role and she should not be expected to take responsibility for informing the family about the patient's significant medical developments. However, (A) remains worse, as you are explicitly disclosing information without patient consent.

2. **D, A, C, E, B**

This question tests your understanding of the consent requirements for different types of procedure. In general, you should only consent a patient for a procedure that you are able to perform by yourself or have sufficient understanding of the risks and benefits to counsel the patient. In this case, a chest drain is an invasive procedure with potentially serious risks and it would be most appropriate to obtain formal written consent (D). The other answers are therefore incorrect; however, the best of these is (A). (A) is better than (C) because a written record is less fallible than human memory, and you may not recall in years to come which nurse witnessed the conversation.

Thorough documentation of consent is always mandatory and has to be the correct answer (D). (E) is clearly wrong, as you are able to consent the patient for this procedure; however, (B) is in some ways worse, as it suggests a complete misunderstanding of what you should do when consenting patients for a relatively simple procedure that you are able to perform.

3. **D, E, B, A, C**

(D) is the best answer, as it is important to adapt to individual patients' disabilities and ensure that they are not disadvantaged simply because a task might become harder. (E) is largely incorrect, although an attempt is being made to obtain a history and there may be useful collateral information in the handover sheet. (B) is a worse option, as no sensible attempt is made at obtaining a history; however, the examination should be sufficient to ensure that the patient is stable, which is your minimum duty in this case. (A) is unnecessary and will not yield any useful information with a profoundly deaf patient if you can communicate this way. (C) is clearly incorrect, as it amounts to doing nothing at all and may disadvantage the patient unnecessarily.

4. C, A, B, D, E

The success of this interview relies on accurate translation of information. For this reason, the best answer which ensures you can communicate effectively with your patient is to arrange an interview with a professional interpreter present (C). The other options are less than ideal, but the next best option is probably (A) to address the brother-in-law directly and insist that he translates word for word what is said, as this may achieve the desired outcome. The difficulty arises because, once doubt has been raised about your ability to trust the brother-in-law's translation, you are then unable to use him as a way of clarifying whether the patient is happy with him translating. (B) is therefore less effective. The difficulty with (D) is that the receptionist speaks a *similar* language to the patient, which introduces another uncertain variable into this already complex scenario. Trying to ascertain the patient's wishes, despite the imperfect conditions of the brother-in-law, is preferable to introducing a third party who may not be able to communicate with the third party at all or may introduce misunderstandings. The worst option is (E), as you are unlikely to find that the consultation either flows or becomes more informative as you attempt communication with a patient who speaks a different language.

5. B, F, H

Although alcohol intake may be pertinent to this elective admission, it can be addressed more effectively after the ward round (B). After your initial assessment, it may be advisable to inform your senior (F) and involve an alcohol services representative (H) if the patient agrees. You should not stop a busy ward round to address non-urgent issues (A) (D), blindly prescribe medication for alcohol withdrawal (C), or give the patient instructions without a full history (E). It would be unprofessional and unhelpful to discourage the nurse from sharing important information (G).

6. A, C, D, E, B

The best answer is to be honest to your colleagues at all times (A). (C) is an unusual, but acceptable, way to approach radiology. It would be better to raise objections directly with your team, but you are being honest as you are not sure what the diagnosis is but are raising the concerns of your seniors and their request for a CT head scan. (D) is less good than (C) because, while still ensuring the scan is done, it will burden your registrar unnecessarily and is unlikely to expedite your scan, as the radiologist will understand the urgency of the indication if you explain the circumstances. The objective should be to obtain the scan as quickly as possible, and (E) will not assist you with your cause in any way. (B) is the worst answer because lying to a colleague can never be justifiable.

7. C, D, E, B, A

It is important that doctors do not routinely work beyond their required hours.

This question is about distinguishing urgent hours which merit working out of hours and routine tasks which are better delegated to a colleague. Therefore, (C) is the best answer. (D) achieves the same goal but is less ideal as the on-call doctor may not be available immediately and urgent tasks may then be delayed. (E) is less ideal for the same reason as (D) in that urgent tasks may be delayed, but in addition a doctor must be asked to review this new patient who has arrived on the ward. (B) is incorrect because jobs are completed based on an arbitrary self-imposed time period, rather than by clinical urgency. The worst option is to make no effort for the patient to be reviewed (A).

8. A, B, F

An apology may help to appease the situation (A), and the opportunity could be used as a learning exercise to obtain feedback on your performance (B). However, you should not be coerced into continuing working in this situation (F), and your only responsibility is to ensure that a thorough and safe handover is completed (E) so that the FY2 doctor can finish the remaining tasks herself (C) (D). It should not be necessary to involve the surgical registrar (G) or consultant (H), unless the situation could not otherwise be resolved.

9. B, C, A, E, D

The correct answer is (B) because a doctor-to-doctor handover will be most likely to ensure that this finding is not missed and clarifies responsibility for following up the result of the interval CT scan. (C) is a less ideal option, as it is less foolproof and places responsibility (perhaps unfairly) on the patient to ensure that interval CT scanning is arranged. However, it is better than (A) which, despite your heroic efforts at highlighting the finding, is likely to be overlooked and could result in the patient being lost to follow-up. Your rheumatology consultant is unlikely to be able to provide the required hospital follow-up this patient may need, and this would be better managed by the GP (E). (D) is the worst answer because it is not the ward clerk's responsibility and they are not sufficiently qualified to undertake this task.

10. B, D, F

As part of your review, you should include the trend in blood results (D), rather than values from a single day (E), which are less informative. You should also document your current management plan (F). As a junior member of the team, you should avoid commenting on the perceived deficits of colleagues (A), unless limiting yourself to factual statements (B). It is not possible to assess a patient retrospectively (C), and notes should only be written retrospectively if this is made very clear. It is never appropriate to avoid documenting your findings (G) and rarely appropriate to undermine colleagues when talking to patients in this way (H).

11. **B, E, H**

Play therapists are a particularly effective resource, as they can invest appropriate time working with children to facilitate successful procedures (B). Before implementing any intervention, it is necessary to explore any concerns of the parents and/or patient and gain their cooperation (E). It is imperative to establish what the patient can comprehend, as learning difficulties span a vast range of cognitive abilities (H). Tricking the patient into the procedure (A) or attempting it in the middle of the night (C) could jeopardize the relationship between clinicians and patient. It would be sensible to attempt options (B), (E), and (H) before resorting to restraints (D) or sedation (F). Inserting a cannula in parents is unnecessary and is unlikely to alleviate the child's concerns (G).

12. **B, C, E, A, D**

A clinician of appropriate experience must consent the patient as usual for her OGD. However, you might be an appropriate person to consent the patient for the additional biopsy and participation in the trial. It is essential that additional consent is obtained, irrespective of her perceived anxieties; therefore, (B) is the correct answer. (C) is a little unclear but is a fairly neutral statement in that you are not told whether the biopsy is going to go ahead or whether you are going to continue seeking consent. It cannot be far wrong to address the patient's anxieties in this way, although obviously it does not directly address the current problem of seeking consent for the biopsy. It is, however, better than (E), which deprives the patient of participating in the trial and potentially weakens the study, but if you feel unable to proceed with the consent process and no one else is available to help, then the patient must be excluded from the study. (A) and (D) are the worst answers; (A) is coercive and seeks to obtain inadequate consent, but this is marginally better than unlawfully removing a biopsy from the patient with no legitimate indication and with no permission from the patient (D).

13. **C, A, B, E, D**

Ensuring a prompt and effective discharge of patients is an important part of being an FY1 doctor. (C) is the best answer as you are being helpful and providing a realistic estimate of the delay before you will be able to complete the discharge letter and have correctly prioritized your unwell patients. (A) is slightly less helpful, as it needlessly involves your registrar who is likely to be busy with other duties. (B) is a further attempt to assist but is a more complex intervention than (C) and (A) and would be more appropriate if clinically urgent commitments were arising together. (E) is less than ideal because it implies that a discharge letter has been rushed and is shorter than it should otherwise be; however, depending on the case, a brief letter may be sufficient to summarize the pertinent aspects of the patient's care. It is certainly preferable to (D) which requires the Ward Sister to complete a duty with which she is likely to be unfamiliar and putting your signature against a document you have not seen.

14. C, A, B, E, D

The key issues here are keeping an open mind while trying to support your colleague. (C) is clearly correct, as there may well be a simple misunderstanding which can be clarified, and you cannot proceed much further without understanding the patient's concerns in detail. (A) is also clearly correct although, in itself, does not offer you the best chance at resolving the issue, as there has been no attempt to understand the complaint in any detail. (B) could represent many different actions, depending on your communication skills and approach to your patient. It may well be appropriate to explain to your patient that the registrar is a very senior doctor and that lung cancer is difficult to tolerate. But this seems unlikely to placate the patient completely and it is probable that some other intervention is also required (e.g. (C) and (A)). (E) and (D) are wrong. The patient has not indicated he has any spiritual questions at the moment or would like to meet a spiritual leader; however, this is perhaps less incorrect than (D), as it is not the role of the FY1 doctor to refer for a treatment which sounds as if your seniors have deemed to be inappropriate.

15. B, E, A, D, C

The correct answer is (B), as it allows you to identify if there are any problems or difficulties that might be impacting on Tim's performance, as well as ensuring he is aware of the developing situation. This is better than (E), as it attempts to resolve the problem itself. (A) is the first incorrect answer, as it fails to address the underlying problem, although it does ensure that the work is completed. (D) and (C) are not constructive suggestions; (D) is unlikely to yield a positive result because of the approach taken, but (C) could easily be interpreted as vindictive, working behind Tim's back, and could result in important tasks going uncompleted.

16. C, D, A, B, E

In any scenario where a colleague voices concerns, you should explore these further to identify ways of alleviating the problem; therefore, (C) is the correct answer. (D) is the next best answer, as it achieves an outcome. The reason that (A) is not better than (D) by itself is that it is a statement of principle and does not resolve the problem at hand. (B) is wrong because you are not in a position to demand that your colleague must perform a particular task, and it is likely to lead to a poor outcome. (E) is the worst answer because it unnecessarily misleads a colleague and exposes them to a health risk.

17. **B, A, D, C, E**

Ward duties must be completed to ensure that patients are safe. In this scenario, you should complete your ward round but postpone any non-urgent discussions until the following day. For this reason, (B) is correct. The other answers are incorrect to various degrees. (A) is the best of these, as it at least allows you to exclude any immediate clinical concerns about the patient, even if it is impolite.

It is difficult to decide between missing your own flight (D) and asking the nurses to remove the families (C), which is impolite. Which of these options is worse will depend on a number of factors. However, it is not without precedent to ask for a few moments alone with a patient, and this is unlikely to cause much distress if done politely. For this reason, it might be preferable to do this than stay late for a non-urgent task and be penalized for doing so by missing your examination.

The worst answer is (E) as by not seeing the patients at all over the course of a day, you could miss their slow deterioration.

18. **C, D, E, A, B**

The GMC guidelines require consent for operations to be taken by someone competent to perform the procedure or an appropriate delegate. The latter must be sufficiently well informed to act as such, and this is likely to exclude FY1 doctors for complex operations such as total knee replacement. The best answer is (C), as in similar questions in other chapters, as you are not sufficiently well informed to counsel a patient thoroughly. All of the remaining answers are wrong, as they involve you obtaining consent for the operation which you must not do. (D) would be the least inappropriate option, as it involves you essentially translating information directly from a suitably qualified person. The next 'best' option might be speaking to the general surgical registrar (E), not because they are able (or likely) to consent the patient, but because they are a senior doctor with experience of the consent process and are likely to set you on the right track, e.g. reminding you that you must not consent the patient for this operation. (A) and (B) are most incorrect because they involve you attempting to directly consent the patient, although (A) is marginally better as you have at least tried to involve a more senior doctor.

19. **A, B, D, C, E**

The best answer is (A). It might be tempting to answer (B) first, as this is naturally the first thing you would do before (A). However, as a single intervention, (A) is more likely to achieve your aim and at least ensures you have discharged the most important aspect of your responsibility to keep the patient informed. (D) seems less likely to solve the problem, as it assumes that the nurses are somehow responsible for his agitation. You have been given no reason in the question to think this might be true.

(C) and (E) are clearly incorrect. (E) is the worst because you cannot choose to treat patients less favourably, based on their lifestyle choices.

20. A, B, C

Death certificates must be completed accurately, as they are a legal record. Senior members of your team (A) (B) are most likely to have a clear idea of the precise cause. A pathologist (C) could help separate multiple complicated circumstances into causes acceptable to the registrar of deaths. The other people listed might contribute under specific circumstances but would not routinely be contacted to establish the cause of death (D) (E) (F) (G) (H).

21. B, C, E, D, A

The minimum you should document in the notes is your findings on examination, and therefore (B) has to be correct. It is better than (C) as, by definition, it offers a more detailed account of your findings than a brief summary. (E) is worse, as documentation should ideally be contemporaneous to ensure maximum accuracy, and you should not usually see other routine cases before writing in the notes for this child. (D) is wrong, as your assessment does not require input from a senior and represents a greater transgression than (E), as your notes should never be modified by anyone else's opinion. The worst answer is (A), as it is opinionated and prejudiced, and you should confine yourself to objective statements and not infer too many details from the parents' appearance.

22. C, B, D, A, E

Documentation is important but must be prioritized after emergencies. You should attend the crash call, even though other doctors will do so, unless another emergency prevents you from going; therefore, (C) is the best answer. (B) is incorrect because, although the immediate life-threatening event is attended to correctly (i.e. the crash call), you return to write in the notes for the fallen patient before attending the next most unwell patient who is febrile. (D) may be judged as worse, as the implication is a complete failure to document clinical encounters in the face of urgent tasks. While it is important to attend crash calls immediately, it would not be prudent to begin deferring or completely avoiding documentation in the notes, as you are asked to see more patients. The implications for (D) are greater than a slight delay in reviewing the febrile patient, and therefore (D) is a worse answer than (B). (A) and (E) are both terribly erroneous, with (A) only being marginally better than (E), as it implies attending to all the other commitments, rather than ignoring the crash call completely (E).

23. B, D, F

You must review the potentially unwell patient as a priority. Doing so with the medical student will provide an extra pair of hands and a valuable learning opportunity (B) (A). The responsibility for reviewing the patient should not be delegated to the student, even if you soon join him (C). You might then ask the student to place the cannula, which should be within his range of experience (D). Although you could site the cannula, this would deprive the student of practice and prevent you from attending to the waiting family (E). You should speak with the patient's family, ideally with a nurse present (F) (G). Although you could speak with the family alone, it is often helpful to have a nursing colleague handy for additional perspective. The family are anticipating a conversation with the medical team and are unlikely to be impressed by a medical student (H).

24. A, F, G

Effective management of trauma requires a rapid multi-disciplinary approach. This is achieved in most hospitals by putting out a trauma call through the switchboard (F). The trauma team will include a general surgeon, an orthopaedic surgeon, an anaesthetist, and emergency physicians. It will also alert ancillary staff (e.g. the on-call radiographer). There should be no additional need to contact the orthopaedic consultant (B). The facts do not suggest major haemorrhage or haematological complications, and so there is not yet a reason to contact the duty haematologist (C).

The trauma team will not routinely include an obstetrician or a neonatologist. Your registrar is contacting obstetrics and so you should contact the neonatology registrar (A). You might also consider sourcing specialist equipment (G) in case an emergency Caesarean section becomes necessary in resuscitation.

The cardiac arrest team will be differently composed to the trauma team (D) and there is no obvious benefit from sourcing phototherapy light (E). Medical students might like to observe if they are present, but given the circumstances, this should not be prioritized (H).

25. B, C, D, E, A

Other colleagues in the hospital will depend on your answering your bleep promptly. However, this must be balanced against the need to complete tasks that you have already started. In this case, it would be unfair to subject the patient to a further needle attempt so you can answer the call, especially now that you have gained access, and so (B) is the correct answer. In attempting (C), you are likely to dislodge the cannula and/or distract your nursing colleagues, and (B) is a simpler option which, if completed, will only lead to a minimal additional delay in answering the bleep. While it is important to do all of the things in (D), after securing the cannula, they can be postponed until you answer the call to avoid further unnecessary delay, and taking longer to answer than in (C). Ignoring the bleep is clearly unacceptable (E) and only marginally better than subjecting the patient to further unnecessary needles (A).

26. B, D, E, C, A

Additional steps should be taken to protect any patient who is particularly anxious about confidentiality. The easiest and most effective step would be to remove sensitive details from your patient list (B). While (D) is also a sensible option, it should already be clear to all healthcare professionals not to disclose clinical information about patients to any family without the patient's consent, although reiteration would not harm the patient.

The patient's confidentiality should be respected like any other patient, but following his request, it may be appropriate to employ added precautions, and therefore (B) and (D) might be considered more appropriate than (E) alone. It is incorrect to coerce the patient into telling his family (C), although you might choose to explore reasons for the patient wanting to keep his diagnosis secret. However, the worst answer is doctoring the medical notes, and this information might be necessary to ensure that he is managed appropriately in future (A).

27. A, B, C, E, D

You have a duty to confront behaviour that threatens patient dignity. As Karen is currently speaking to the child in a way that you think is inappropriate, you should raise the issue immediately, and therefore (A) is the best answer. You may wish to approach the nursing hierarchy, instead of speaking to Karen directly (B), although this would be a more appropriate first step if the behaviour causing you concern had already happened (as opposed to currently happening). It is incorrect to attempt to investigate Karen's behaviour by talking to other staff (C), which might be seen as gossip or bullying. However, gaining additional corroboratory evidence in this way is probably less extreme than informing officials in the Trust at this stage; from the scenario description, it would seem fair to escalate concerns within the ward hierarchy before doing so anywhere else (E). It is clearly never appropriate to ignore this issue, and once you have developed a concern, it should always be acted upon in a way that satisfies you that the issue will not arise again (D).

28. C, B, D, A, E

The most sensible immediate course of action is (C). This may allow you to facilitate immediate improvements, and you might discover that the patient is more interested in communicating her concerns than making a formal complaint per se. It may become apparent that the patient should be directed to PALS (B) which will offer her a formal route through which to lodge her complaint, but this is a less ideal immediate course of action, and (C) may resolve the concerns with greater expediency. While the consultant should be informed that the patient is considering making a complaint (D), in order to facilitate a discussion between them and the patient, it is a less appropriate response to the patient than responding to her query and providing her the option of PALS. The patient should never be discouraged from lodging a complaint (A), but perhaps marginally worse than dissuading the patient is inciting them to generate a complaint that you believe is necessary (E)—instead your own concerns should be raised openly with the senior team.

29. A, B, F

Patient safety is always your priority and this patient should be saved an unnecessary catheterization (A) (D).

Although you are the responsible clinician in this case, you cannot accept full responsibility for the error (G). The student is not yet a doctor, but he must take some responsibility for any procedures he performs. He should have checked the patient's identity and indication before proceeding. For this reason, both you and the student should apologize to the misidentified patient (F). However, it would be unfair to blame the student entirely, and mistakes are best learnt from by helping to rectify the consequences, not by being sent home (C).

A clinical incident form should then be completed (B) to create a paper trail and in case lessons can be learnt for the future. You should identify any contributing factors, e.g. a patient in the wrong bed or not wearing a wristband. You should certainly not mislead the patient (E), and there is no clinical indication for an ultrasound KUB (H).

30. A, E, B, C, D

The patient requiring scrotal exploration needs to be consented promptly, so that he can be taken to theatre. However, GMC guidance clearly states that the person taking consent should usually be able to perform the procedure themselves. In this case, your registrar is the most appropriate person to take consent once they are available (A). Clearly it is less ideal to involve someone else outside of care of this patient but (E) does offer a reasonable solution. The consultant would have enough experience to consent the patient, but contacting him at home is unlikely to persuade him to come in for this purpose and is unlikely to reflect best on your own abilities to resolve this matter with more practicable solutions discussed earlier (B). (C) is in fact useless, as the medical registrar is unlikely to offer advice beyond telling you not to take the consent yourself. (D), however, is the worst answer, as an incorrect consent can amount to negligence if an issue were to arise afterwards.

31. B, C, E

Although the man's tape recorder and aggressive tone apply pressure, you should remain resilient and adhere to the general principles of professionalism.

You should try to ignore the tape recorder (B) and explain that you cannot discuss a patient's care without their consent (C) (F). If he persists and/or is threatening, you might like to ask him to leave and contact security if necessary (E).

Saying 'no comment' is unhelpful (A), as is passing the problem on to a colleague (D) who is unlikely to appreciate the gesture. You should certainly not lie to the relative (G), despite his aggressive tone, or exacerbate the situation by attempting to turn off the tape recorder (H).

32. D, E, B, A, C

Although you are with medical students, this should not stop you exercising compassion when one of your patients is visibly upset. You should leave the students at a distance and ascertain what has happened to lower his mood, and therefore (D) is the most appropriate action. While (E) implies you are raising the topic of whether he would feel comfortable with the teaching session, it ignores the patient's current emotional state. It seems unfair to trivialize the patient's emotional state (B) into a teaching point for the students, and this still does not immediately address whether he wishes to continue with the teaching session. However, this is probably still fairer than asking the patient to assist with student teaching earlier, and then not giving him the opportunity to choose (A). It is imperative to give the patient a choice, and worse than not offering is insisting, ignoring his crying, and continuing with the teaching session, as this is likely to be awkward for your students and potentially further upsetting for the patient (C).

33. A, E, F

You should listen to Meredith and try to understand her perspective (A) before talking her through the procedure again, with reference to any specific concerns she might have expressed (E). If there is a possibility that she might opt to cancel the procedure, you should speak with your registrar early (F). She might benefit from counselling by a more senior doctor, and cancellations are best anticipated early in case other patients can fill the operating slot. However, you should not coerce the patient's decision (G) or make light of the operation that she is worried about (H). Patient concerns about an operation fall squarely within your remit, and the nursing staff should not be discouraged from contacting you about similar problems in future (B). Speaking to the patient's family (D) or referring her to a psychologist (C) would be presumptuous, as you do not know whether this is what she would want.

34. B, D, A, C, E

Ideally, any explanation should start by finding out what your audience already knows, and therefore (B) is the best answer. This prevents repetition of knowledge and allows you to clarify any specific misunderstandings. It is also often helpful to provide patient information leaflets (D) for patients to read in their own time; however, this is somewhat less sensitive as a first measure and does not offer any opportunity for a two-way discussion; they are best used as an adjunct to verbal explanation, so that patients have an opportunity to ask questions. Although heart failure is inability of the pump to perfuse the tissues (A), this textbook definition might be lost on a patient hearing it for the first time and is probably less helpful than providing a pamphlet written for patients. However, this accurate description is probably preferable to an over-simplification (C) which can sound frightening, and you should beware of letting patients who present with occasional ankle swelling go home thinking that you have diagnosed a terminal illness. Although Stephen should read about heart failure if he wishes, patients can easily become lost in the masses of information available online, and therefore the least helpful advice is to recommend this as the first source of information; hence, (E) is the worst answer.

35. A, B, F

It is important to share information with patients, but only if this is what they want. We should not force information on them any more than we should force anything else. However, you do have a duty to make sure that Rachel understands why it would be helpful to her to talk about her disease (A). You should try to understand her perspective by listening carefully (B). If she continues to choose not to know, the issue should not be raised again unless there is reason to think that she has changed her mind (F).

You should certainly not coerce her to accept information by providing written leaflets (D) or asking other team members to approach the subject (G) (H). If Rachel consents, you could talk to her family, but in the absence of such an agreement, they should not be told anything more than normal (C). It would be callous to obstruct Rachel's happiness by telling her that she should be otherwise (E).

36. D, A, B, E, C

Your seniors are better placed to attend this meeting (D), as they will know the patient and might already have a rapport with Jenny. They will also have greater experience with conversations of this nature. The next best option if you do attend the meeting is to familiarize yourself with the patient's notes beforehand (A). Asking the nurse to brief you would be inadequate preparation for such an important meeting, and therefore (B) is less appropriate. Even less appropriate would be attempting to identify the issues as the conversation unfolds (E). The worst answer is (C), as it would be unhelpful and awkward for all parties if you attended the meeting but declined to contribute.

37. B, C, E, A, D

You should learn from previous mistakes, whether your own or a colleague's. You will want to let your registrar know that errors have occurred in this way previously, and therefore (B) is the best response. He might then amend his strategy or decide that the investigation is sufficiently urgent to proceed with the original plan. (C) represents a less foolproof mechanism of booking the scan but should also lead to the correct imaging being performed. Although it may be preferable for the registrar to take responsibility for requesting the scan (E), this is unlikely to foster a good working relationship between you, and you are still failing to address the issue of mistaken imaging requests being submitted. It is clearly less preferable to attempt to establish contact with radiology after making the imaging request, as this increases the likelihood that the request will be processed incorrectly (A). (D) is the worst response, as it would not be a measured response to complete a clinical incident form.

38. A, B, C, E, D

In this unenviable position, you are nevertheless duty-bound to raise your concern and should do so with the operating surgeon (A). The scrub nurse should certainly recount the swabs, but this instruction might be better coming from the surgeon himself; therefore, (B) is less ideal.

Many studies of human error have found that juniors are too indirect when questioning more experienced colleagues. If you believe that a swab might have been left in the abdomen, you should say so, and asking other questions first is likely to try your consultant's patience when a direct question would have been sufficient (C). (E) is similarly unfavourable and perhaps more irritating (and therefore may be worse). However, clearly the worst option would be to remain quiet, as you might have been the only person with the opportunity to stop the patient undergoing a second operation to remove an aberrant swab (D).

39. D, B, E, C, A

Finding people who are sufficiently senior to complete work-based assessments can be difficult. However, these are useful learning experiences and a minimum number are necessary to pass FY1. The Foundation Programme is 'trainee-led' which means that you are responsible for finding sufficient learning opportunities and assessors to complete the minimum number. For this reason, you should remind the consultant who promised you a work-based assessment (D). The next option (B) is less ideal, as it also involves you discussing more cases with that individual who might not have the time or opportunity for. It would only be after attempting both these strategies that you might consider informing your Educational Supervisor (E), but to do so before would be premature and inefficient. The foundation school is unlikely to be interested at that time, and therefore (C) is a less ideal option. Of course, it would be dishonest to masquerade as your consultant and complete the assessment yourself, and therefore the worst answer is (A).

40. C, D, E, B, A

Management plans change with time according to new information, evolving clinical signs, and the approach of the clinicians involved. It is important that doctors—and particularly consultants—have discretion in managing patients.

However, you should point out the discrepancy between the two plans (C), as this might make the second consultant consider why they differ. It would only be if he insists that you should generally implement his plan as he is now ultimately responsible for the patient, but clearly (D) would be less preferred to (C). (E) risks undermining the consultant by seeking an uninvited third opinion. If you have serious concerns about a new management plan, you should of course raise these and take necessary action to avoid harm occurring. If you are uncertain, your registrar might be able to explain the reason for this new approach. Clarifying to whom you are ultimately responsible might be interpreted as impertinent (B)—you are clinically accountable to the consultant on duty that day, and therefore (B) is probably marginally more unprofessional than (E). (A) is likely to be slightly worse than (E), as the implication here is that the consultant simply needs to see the patient in order for his management plan to be followed. Although it would be sensible to ask the consultant to see Mr Smith, you should not coerce him to do so by refusing to implement his plan otherwise (A). It is pragmatic to accept that senior doctors will not always review patients before instigating a management plan.

41. C, E, G

The scenario requires you to balance the training needs of you and your colleagues with the service demands on your seniors. As part of FY1, you are expected to receive appropriate teaching (A) (B), and this is not necessarily interchangeable with personal preparation for your chosen specialist exams (F). Options (C) and (E) best seek to resolve the problem while being proactive and not relying simply on other colleagues (H), although escalation (e.g. through your Foundation Programme Director) might be necessary at some stage. Recording the feedback in an end-of-placement survey will allow the feedback to be formally recorded and may result in changes for future trainees. It is less ideal than (C) and (E) by itself as an option, as it cannot change things for the current crop of foundation doctors. If you do approach a senior colleague, it is likely to be your Clinical Supervisor or Educational Supervisor. The Medical Director has overall responsibility for doctors in the hospital and so is unlikely to be an appropriate person to contact at an early stage.

42. A, C, F

In the event of a serious allegation, it might be necessary to explore a complaint in further detail and involve yourself to a greater extent than is suggested by this scenario. However, in this case, no issues have been raised that might cause you a moral obligation to become further involved. It would probably be correct to exempt yourself from the situation (F). It would be reasonable to ask a close friend for further information (A) and reasonable to offer non-specific advice about hospital complaints systems (C). It would be unwise to become any further involved, e.g. by talking directly to the consultant concerned (B), attempting to suppress a potential complaint (G), or interfering with the delivery of your friend's healthcare (H). As you should not be involved in the situation to any great extent, there should not be a reason to involve any third parties, e.g. your employer (E) or medical defence organization (D).

43. A, D, C, B, E

It is clearly important to establish what the patient/family member understands already, otherwise you might risk obfuscating the situation further (A). Option (D) is also a good answer, as it sounds as if a strong grasp of the situation will be necessary before proceeding further. It comes a very close second, as (A) will also help the patient's wife feel as if her concerns are being addressed as well as providing important background information.

Your registrar may enable them to offer further insights, but this step might be unnecessary if you can understand what has happened from the patient's wife and medical notes (C). Option (B) might be necessary in some cases, but it is likely that you will be able to resolve a number of misunderstandings yourself. If this were not the case, arranging contact with the patient's responsible consultant would be an early next step (B). Referring the patient's wife to the hospital complaints team is premature at this stage and does not attempt to address her concerns (E).

44. D, E, H

It is important to establish whether there is in fact any problem, and therefore asking the patient afterwards if he has any questions about the procedure would allow you to establish whether the communication difficulties you perceived were genuine (E). You could speak with the consultant to ask if he thinks the patient understood everything (H), and option (D) would allow you to feed back any concerns about communication or consent to senior staff within the department. Further independent investigations into patient safety, involving ancillary staff, and looking into professional qualifications are outside of your scope (B) (F) (G). Immigration authorities (C) do not have a role to play in this case.

45. D, A, C, B, E

The best solution is to explain to the patient that leaving hospital is in his interest (D), as this could result in an amicable solution. Option (A) might also be necessary but is less ideal than (D), as it attempts to achieve the same result but indirectly via the patient's family. It is likely that you will need to begin his discharge paperwork, but completing this does not solve the problem in and of itself (C). (B) is clearly incorrect, as patients should not be able to remain in hospital inappropriately simply because they are upset. However, calling security does not address the patient's unwillingness to leave and is likely to exacerbate the problem further. If security were to be involved in a patient's routine departure from hospital, this would take place at the end of a very long process and would not usually be initiated by a foundation doctor.

Patient focus

Introduction

As a junior doctor, you are constantly pulled in different directions by multiple competing interests. These include those of your immediate bosses (possibly multiple consultants, a registrar, and an SHO), Educational Supervisors (Clinical Supervisor, Foundation Programme Director), fellow FY1 doctors, other healthcare professionals (nurses, physiotherapists), ancillary services (laboratory, radiology), patients' relatives, representatives of the Trust (infection control, human resources, information technology), and many others. In amongst all of these is a patient, if not many, for whom all of these individuals are also working.

It will not come as a surprise that *Good Medical Practice* (2013) states early on that you must 'make the care of your patient your first concern' and 'treat patients as individuals and respect their dignity'. In addition, *Good Medical Practice* requires that you:

- listen to, and respond to, their concerns and preferences
- give patients the information they want or need in a way they can understand
- respect patients' right to reach decisions with you about their treatment and care
- support patients in caring for themselves to improve and maintain their health.

Refusal of lifesaving treatment

One challenge is when patients reach decisions that are contrary to the best available medical advice. The archetypal case in point is that of a Jehovah's Witness at risk of life-threatening haemorrhage but refusing a blood transfusion. In such cases, remember that:

- you should never assume what someone's beliefs are just because they come bearing a particular religious label. It is always right to ask the patient what *they* believe and what *they* will accept under different circumstances. For example, some Jehovah's Witnesses will accept cell salvage and some blood substitutes
- seek advice early, particularly if the stakes are high (e.g. active bleeding). Your own seniors (SpR, consultant, etc.) and the on-call haematology team are good places to start. They may direct you to other resources that you might contact (with the patient's consent) such as the Jehovah's Witnesses' Hospital Liaison Committee
- document all conversations (with the patient and colleagues) carefully

- ultimately, an adult patient with capacity has the right to refuse treatments—however much you disagree and even if this ultimately results in their death. It should go without saying that such cases will not be managed by you alone as a foundation doctor!

Decision-making and capacity

A much more common scenario that you will encounter during the Foundation Programme is the need to make decisions about patients who are unable to make decisions for themselves. The Mental Capacity Act 2005 lays down a number of principles, which include:

- Everyone has a right to make their own decisions. A patient should be presumed to have capacity unless it is shown (through a capacity assessment) that this is not the case.
- All efforts should be made to help patients make decisions for themselves, e.g. by providing information in a different format or waiting until they regain capacity if the delay will not cause them harm.
- A patient should not be assumed to lack capacity just because the decision they are making is unwise or against medical advice.

The Mental Capacity Act 2005 states that a patient is deemed to be lacking capacity at a particular time and for a specific decision if they:

- have an 'impairment of, or a disturbance in the functioning of, the mind or brain' **and** are unable to
- understand the information relevant to the decision,
- retain that information,
- use or weigh that information as part of the process of making the decision, **or**
- communicate his decision (whether by talking, using sign language, or any other means).

In such cases, the responsible clinician should make decisions for the patient, but this must be in their 'best interests'. In doing so, the decision-maker must consider:

- the person's past and present wishes and feelings,
- the beliefs and values that would be likely to influence the decision if he had capacity, and
- the views of anyone named by the person as someone to be consulted, engaged in caring for the person or interested in his welfare, any donee of a lasting power of attorney granted by the person, and any deputy appointed for the person by the court.

Answering questions in this domain

Questions within this section assess your ability to keep the patient as the focus of care at all times. To achieve this, you should listen carefully to patients' ideas, concerns, and expectations, and understand that their needs often go beyond a 'positive clinical outcome'. You should always show compassion and respect while working with patients, to develop a management plan that suits their needs.

- Patient safety is your first priority, always.
- Patient safety is only part of your responsibility. You should also look out for patients' dignity, convenience, and general well-being.
- Work with patients when developing a treatment plan. Understand their perspective, and then communicate yours clearly.
- Doctors and other healthcare professionals can contribute to the well-being of patients beyond simply treating disease. Good health is a consequence of biomedical, psychological, and social factors.

References and further reading

Francis R (2013). *The Mid Staffordshire NHS Foundation Trust Public Inquiry*. If you have the time, it is worth reading through selected parts of the *Francis Report* (2013) into the scandal at Stafford Hospital in which it is alleged that there was an organizational loss of patient focus. There are lessons in this report that could be learnt by all doctors and aspiring healthcare leaders.

General Medical Council (2013). *Good Medical Practice*. http://www.gmc-uk.org/guidance/good_medical_practice/professionalism_in_action.asp

Mental Capacity Act 2005. http://www.legislation.gov.uk/ukpga/2005/9/contents

QUESTIONS

1. Mavis has recently been widowed and has a history of mild dementia. She was admitted several weeks ago with pneumonia, which has gradually resolved. She worked hard with the physiotherapy team and has returned to her functional baseline level of activity. Despite this, her family highlights several concerns which the nurses are keen for you to address before Mavis is discharged.

Rank in order the following actions in response to this situation (1 = Most appropriate; 5 = Least appropriate)

A Assist Mavis's daughter-in-law, who feels that Mavis requires a lot of help with looking after her bungalow.

B Address her son's concerns about possible financial exploitation by a neighbour, using the appropriate assessment tools.

C Address her brother's concerns that her memory loss is becoming much worse and she needs further medical treatment.

D Discuss the family's concerns with Mavis, and obtain her perspective first.

E Assist the nephew who has asked you to arrange a nursing home for Mavis, where she can be supervised, in case she falls.

2. You have arranged some bedside teaching for a group of six medical students with a patient on your ward who is suffering from multiple sclerosis. On arrival, you find her to be in emotional distress due to worsening of symptoms and a recent financial dispute with her family. You had previously agreed to spend 45 minutes with the patient and students, and do not have any other patient with whom you could teach the students.

Rank in order the following actions in response to this situation (1 = Most appropriate; 5 = Least appropriate)

A Teach the students clinical theory in a classroom instead.

B Explain that emotional turbulence is a normal part of chronic disease, and continue with the bedside teaching as planned.

C Attempt teaching, but agree that if she continues to be upset, you are happy to discontinue.

D Teach the students a lesson in communication skills by exploring her family issues.

E Ignore the issue altogether, and restrict your teaching to brief examination of the patient's neurological system.

3. You are a foundation doctor working in a GP surgery and have spent the morning assessing an infant with possible meningitis, admitting a young man with suicidal ideation, and breaking the news of a pancreatic malignancy to a previously healthy 55-year-old. Prior to your lunchtime home visits, a 60-year-old man visits your practice for the fourth time in two months with generalized worsening 'aches', despite normal examination, investigations, and maximal medical therapy. Your ten-minute consultation fails to assuage him.

Rank in order the following actions in response to this situation (1 = Most appropriate; 5 = Least appropriate)

A Explain that you must see other patients with serious life-threatening conditions, and you do not have the time he requires.

B Ask whether he would be interested in the services of complementary health providers.

C Refer the patient to a rheumatologist.

D Spend ten minutes focusing on the patient's psychological and social well-being.

E Offer the patient the advice of another doctor at the practice.

4. A patient appears to be worried during your surgical ward round, and the consultant suggests the need to 'get to the bottom of these worries before we explore the different treatment options'. You consider how you might go about doing this.

Rank in order the following actions in response to this situation (1 = Most appropriate; 5 = Least appropriate)

A Allow the patient to express their concerns when they choose and without directly asking.

B Ask the nurse looking after the patient today to explore any concerns.

C Ask the healthcare assistant (HCA) looking after the patient today to explore any concerns.

D Speak to the family to identify any concerns that the patient may have.

E Set aside 20 minutes to speak with the patient to establish any underlying concerns.

5. One of your patients appears to be very depressed, which she believes to have been precipitated by a recent bereavement. You realize that her loss parallels one of your own experiences and wonder how this might be used to develop rapport with your patient.

Rank in order the following actions in response to this situation (1 = Most appropriate; 5 = Least appropriate)

A Describe your own loss and subsequent feelings in detail.

B Explain how you can empathize with her because of your own similar loss.

C Acknowledge her understandable sadness from experiencing a personal loss.

D Change the subject, as dwelling on it may make her more upset.

E Encourage her to discuss her feelings with a friend, family member, or religious leader.

6. You are working as an FY1 doctor on the gastroenterology ward. Maureen has early dementia and declines further treatment, despite the medical team's recommendations and her daughter's insistence. Her daughter explains about a previous protracted debate between other doctors and her mother, which led to Maureen eventually being 'overruled', and asks you to avoid a similar delay and initiate treatment straightaway.

Rank in order the following actions in response to this situation (1 = Most appropriate; 5 = Least appropriate)

A Assess Maureen's capacity for refusing this treatment.

B Read through the notes and establish whether Maureen lacks capacity.

C Ask the daughter to help in your assessment of Maureen's capacity.

D Just get on and treat Maureen, irrespective of her wishes.

E Avoid the decision and seek the input of a superior.

7. You are seeing Derek, a 45-year-old man. He specifically mentions to you his relative who has recently been diagnosed with cancer. This news has concerned him, and Derek is worried about his own risk of developing cancer. Having done some reading on the Internet, he is requesting a full-body CT scan.

Rank in order the following actions in response to this situation (1 = Most appropriate; 5 = Least appropriate)

A Explain the dangers of X-radiation and the associated increased risk for cancer.

B Explain that his absolute risk of developing cancer is low.

C Take a history and examination.

D Offer a full-body CT scan.

E Prescribe anxiolytics.

8. You are reviewing a man who is troubled about his weight. Despite having tried various dieting and exercise plans, he is now requesting medication for weight loss. His body mass index (BMI) is currently 35, and under local policy guidelines, he has not yet reached the BMI required to commence this treatment.

Rank in order the following actions in response to this situation (1 = Most appropriate; 5 = Least appropriate)

A Write him a prescription, as he has exhausted alternative options.

B Explain the high cost of this medication, and encourage him to seek it from wholesale online distributors instead.

C Write to the Clinical Commissioning Group (CCG), asking permission to prescribe the medication.

D Inform the patient that he is not of a high enough weight to benefit sufficiently from the medication.

E Refer the patient to another doctor in the practice.

9. You are asked by one of the nursing staff to see Heather, a patient who is refusing elective coronary angiography following a non-ST elevation myocardial infarction.

Rank in order the following actions in response to this situation (1 = Most appropriate; 5 = Least appropriate)

A Establish her concerns.

B Take the patient to see a coronary angiography being performed.

C Discuss her decision with family members if Heather agrees.

D Explore alternative treatment options, and their risks and benefits.

E Explain the benefits of the procedure, and insist that she must have it done.

10. You are about to share a list of ward jobs after the consultant ward round with your SHO on the oncology ward. You both have plenty of tasks to keep you busy until the end of your shift. The SHO tells you to delay referring Mrs Wilson to the palliative care team until tomorrow, as she is likely to need infusion pumps and will create other tasks which will take too long. You are concerned as she seems to be in pain.

Rank in order the following actions in response to this situation (1 = Most appropriate; 5 = Least appropriate)

A Complete the list of jobs that your SHO has assigned to you before referring the patient to the palliative care team at the end of the day.

B Delegate the task of referring the patient to a nurse, although you know that 'doctor-to-doctor' referrals are expected.

C Complain to your consultant that the SHO is neglecting Mrs Wilson.

D Explain the importance of adequate analgesia in terminal patients to your SHO, and suggest that the jobs be reprioritized.

E Follow your colleague's instructions, and make the referral to the palliative care team tomorrow.

11. You are working in a genitourinary medicine clinic. A patient attends because she believes that she may have contracted an infection following a recent sexual encounter outside of her long-term relationship.

Choose the THREE most appropriate actions to take in this situation

A Advise her to begin contact tracing, i.e. informing her regular partner.

B Suggest you will have to inform her long-term partner if she does not.

C Test for HIV as HIV testing is mandatory.

D Advise a blood test for syphilis antibody.

E Promote safe sexual practices.

F Discuss the morality of multiple sexual partners.

G Inform the patient's GP to ensure adequate community follow-up.

H Ask a phlebotomist to draw the blood sample to avoid the risk of a needle-stick injury.

12. You have arrived on a ward to review a medical outlier. You retrieve the patient's notes from the treatment room after several wasted minutes searching for them in the notes trolley. You are exasperated as you risk missing lunch, again, if not en route to the canteen within ten minutes. The telephone at the nurses' station rings. There is no ward clerk. Although the surgical FY1 doctor and his registrar, a staff nurse, and a physiotherapist are standing at the desk, no one answers after 20 rings.

Choose the THREE most appropriate actions to take in this situation

A Tell the surgical FY1 doctor to answer the phone.

B Tell the staff nurse that you are in a great hurry and that she/he should answer the phone.

C Move away from the nurses' station quickly, and let the phone be answered by someone else.

D Ask the staff nurse whether you can answer the phone, and let her/him know what is needed.

E Pick up the phone, and give the handset straight to the staff nurse saying 'It's for you'.

F Ask people at the desk whether someone is waiting for a call, and answer the phone if no one volunteers.

G Ask the nurse in charge whether there is a policy on answering phones on the ward.

H State to all around the desk that the call might be very important for a relative/carer or directly related to patient care.

13. During your first month working on the neurosurgery ward, you have become increasingly troubled by your registrar's ability. You have seen him misinterpret basic clinical signs. On one occasion, you tried to share your concerns with the consultant in charge, but he discounted them, highlighting the registrar's natural ability in the operating room.

Rank in order the following actions in response to this situation (1 = Most appropriate; 5 = Least appropriate)

A Ask your consultant again to consider the registrar's overall performance.

B Inform your Educational Supervisor.

C Approach the registrar, and ask him whether he would be willing to receive teaching from you after work.

D Inform the Clinical Director.

E Share your thoughts with another FY1 colleague.

14. You are the paediatric FY1 doctor. A nurse asks if you could speak with the family of a 13-year-old patient, Lenka, who does not speak any English. Lenka's family is very angry, and they demand that she is moved away from the neighbouring patient who has been coughing vigorously throughout the night. You also notice that Lenka appears to be upset.

Choose the THREE most appropriate actions to take in this situation

A Acknowledge the family's concern, and try to move the patient into a side room.

B Explain to the patient's family the low risk of contracting an infection from neighbouring patients in open bays on the ward.

C Try to establish Lenka's concerns.

D Try to address the concerns of Lenka's family first.

E Ask the neighbouring patient if they would be willing to move into a side room.

F Provide the patient and her family with face masks.

G Ask the ward nurse to address these nursing concerns.

H Provide the neighbouring patient with a face mask.

15. You are clerking patients in the Medical Admissions Unit (MAU). A former colleague approaches and informs you that his father is one of the patients waiting to be clerked. He asks you to see his father first.

Rank in order the following actions in response to this situation (1 = Most appropriate; 5 = Least appropriate)

A Report your medical colleague to his Educational Supervisor.

B Refuse your colleague's request outright.

C Ask the registrar whether he has any preference for which patient you should see next and, if not, begin with your colleague's father.

D See your colleague's father last, as punishment for his unfair request.

E Establish if there is any particular reason why he wants you to see his father straightaway.

16. Lucy is a 24-year-old with Crohn's disease. On reviewing her drug chart, you find that multiple doses of medication have not been given. On questioning the nurse who has been looking after Lucy since her admission, she says that the patient has been refusing to take the medication when offered. However, you have always found the patient to be pleasant and cooperative. Lucy denies being offered any medication by the nurse.

Rank in order the following actions in response to this situation (1 = Most appropriate; 5 = Least appropriate)

A Report the nurse to the Royal College of Nursing.

B File a clinical incident form for failing to satisfactorily encourage Lucy to take her medication.

C Suggest that the nurse sits with Lucy and encourages her to take her medication.

D Change all her medication to intravenous forms.

E Inform the ward sister that Lucy has not been receiving her medications, and ask her to investigate further.

17. Mr Stevenson has recently been diagnosed with terminal meso-thelioma. During his admission for a chest infection, you are handed an indefinite DNACPR (Do Not Attempt Cardio-Pulmonary Resuscitation) order that has been in place since a previous admission. On speaking to Mr Stevenson and his family, they do not appear to be aware that this order is in place.

Rank in order the following actions in response to this situation (1 = Most appropriate; 5 = Least appropriate)

A Tear up the DNACPR order.

B Explain the futility of cardiopulmonary resuscitation in Mr Stevenson's case as the logic of the DNACPR order.

C Apologize for the insufficient explanation given by Mr Stevenson's previous clinicians.

D Inform your registrar immediately.

E Do not inform Mr Stevenson and his family about the DNACPR order at this time, but wait to discuss the matter with Mr Stevenson alone.

18. You are taking a history from the mother of 11-year-old Clara who has presented with shoulder pain. When you are left alone with Clara, she admits that her mother often gets upset with her and has occasionally hit her in the past. The mother has appeared completely appropriate in her interaction with Clara.

Rank in order the following actions in response to this situation (1 = Most appropriate; 5 = Least appropriate)

A Clara is most likely referring to reasonable chastisement, and the issue should not be pursued.

B Confront Clara's mother about the accusation, and ask her to volunteer any explanations.

C Document the comments clearly, and attempt to gain more information from Clara, alone if possible.

D Begin a thorough head-to-toe examination of Clara once her mother has returned and, if asked, explain that you are looking for bruises.

E Inform the police.

19. You are about to discharge Terence following his admission for treatment for recurrent epileptic seizures. On getting up to leave the bedside, you overhear his wife's surprise at the doctors allowing him to return to work as a heavy goods vehicle driver. You feel sure that Terence has no intention of relinquishing his driving responsibilities, despite promises to the contrary.

Rank in order the following actions in response to this situation (1 = Most appropriate; 5 = Least appropriate)

A Seek assurances from Terence's wife that he will not return to work.

B Inform Terence's GP.

C Ask Terence to sign an agreement not to return to work in the medical notes.

D Disclose his diagnosis to the Driver and Vehicle Licensing Agency (DVLA).

E You are not responsible for the patient's actions once you have appropriately instructed him.

20. A 40-year-old mother of two children stops you as you are walking by her side room and asks to speak with you. She is visibly worried about the results of her pancreatic biopsy and asks, 'What will happen if I have cancer?'

Rank in order the following actions in response to this situation (1 = Most appropriate; 5 = Least appropriate)

A Reassure the patient that the medical team will do everything they can to try to treat her.

B Reassure her that everything will be fine.

C Ask the patient to wait and ask your senior any questions.

D Echo her concern: 'I can see that you are worried that you might have cancer.'

E Do not say anything, but instead look away in an effort to communicate the grave nature of her problem non-verbally.

21. Iris is 87 and one of your patients on the care of the elderly ward. She has mild dementia but tells you that she does not like being dressed by the nursing staff each morning. At home, her carer just stands by in case she needs help, although she concedes that this 'takes longer' than allowing the carer to dress her.

Rank in order the following actions in response to this situation (1 = Most appropriate; 5 = Least appropriate)

A Tell Iris that as soon as she goes home, she will be able to go back to her old routine.

B Tell Iris that she can dress herself each morning if she prefers, with help if necessary.

C Pass on Iris's request to the ward sister, and ask that it be passed on during the nursing handover.

D Explain that this is probably not possible as the nursing staff are busiest in the mornings.

E Tell Iris that you cannot interfere with how the ward is run.

22. You are asked by the nurses to site a urethral catheter for Arthur who is an elderly man who needs to urinate frequently. He has known prostate trouble and reduced mobility. It takes at least five minutes to get him to the toilet, after which he often does not need to urinate after all.

Rank in order the following actions in response to this situation (1 = Most appropriate; 5 = Least appropriate)

A Ask Arthur for his views and whether he is troubled about multiple visits to the toilet.

B Offer other options such as a commode or a male external catheter.

C Speak to the urology team to ask if there is anything further that can be done to minimize Arthur's lower urinary tract symptoms.

D Explain the problem to Arthur and then insert a urethral catheter once he consents.

E Tell Arthur that he needs a urethral catheter and then site it carefully.

23. You arrive on the ward one morning to find a student nurse washing a male patient with the curtains open. The patient does not appear to be obviously concerned.

Rank in order the following actions in response to this situation (1 = Most appropriate; 5 = Least appropriate)

A Pull the curtains closed.

B Ask the patient for his preference and leave the curtains open if he chooses.

C Explain the need to ensure patient privacy to the student nurse afterwards if she is unclear.

D Tell the student nurse in front of the patient that she should learn to respect privacy.

E Carry on with your job as there is not a problem and you should not interfere.

24. You are on a fast-paced surgical ward round. Your consultant tells a patient that she will need a 'Hartmann's procedure which will leave a colostomy' and she signs a consent form. You can tell from her body language that she wants to ask questions but does not feel able to do so.

Rank in order the following actions in response to this situation (1 = Most appropriate; 5 = Least appropriate)

A Explain that you will come back after the ward round in case she wants to ask any more questions.

B Insist that the consultant stays until he has answered her questions.

C Tell the patient that your consultant will come back later to answer questions.

D Let the ward round continue, but remain behind to draw a picture for the patient illustrating the Hartmann's procedure.

E Continue with the ward round, but return later to answer questions.

25. As you are sitting at the nurses' station completing a discharge summary, you see a 55-year-old patient walking away from you with his gown flapping open at the back.

Rank in order the following actions in response to this situation (1 = Most appropriate; 5 = Least appropriate)

A Shout to the patient by name so that he can be alerted to his state of undress.

B Catch up with the patient and let him know that he is partially undressed.

C Help him tie up the gown correctly.

D Find a nurse and let them know the patient needs assistance.

E Catch up with the patient and tell him that he should be more careful in case he embarrasses other patients or visitors.

26. Your Trust occasionally authorizes use of protective mittens for certain patients. These are large gloves that essentially prevent patients from using their hands. You are asked to prescribe mittens for a patient out of hours and agree to do so only under specific conditions.

Rank in order the following actions in response to this situation (1 = Most appropriate; 5 = Least appropriate)

A The patient is confused.

B The patient lacks capacity.

C The patient lacks capacity and is at risk of pulling out essential lines and tubes.

D The patient lacks capacity and has pulled out lines and tubes, and alternative strategies have been unsuccessful.

E The patient lacks capacity and is at risk of pulling out essential lines and tubes. The patient's next of kin are fiercely opposed to the use of mittens.

27. A patient admitted to your ward with pneumonia is shown to have tuberculosis (TB). He is asked to wear a face mask when he leaves his side room and is told that the case must be reported to the Health Protection Agency (HPA). He refuses to allow information about his illness to be sent externally and is often seen outside his side room without a mask.

Rank in order the following actions in response to this situation (1 = Most appropriate; 5 = Least appropriate)

A Explore the reasons for this patient's non-compliance.

B Explain that TB is potentially dangerous and very easily spread to others in the hospital.

C Explain that you will not send his details externally but that his GP must be informed.

D Explain to the patient, but submit his details to the Health Protection Agency (HPA), regardless of whether he gives consent.

E Discharge the patient from hospital without further treatment as he is a danger to other patients.

28. Ron is an elderly man with bowel obstruction. He is delirious and keeps pulling out intravenous cannulae, as well as occasionally tugging on his nasogastric tube. Reinserting cannulae is becoming increasingly time-consuming and he is running out of suitable veins.

Rank in order the following actions in response to this situation (1 = Most appropriate; 5 = Least appropriate)

A Resite cannulae in areas less likely to be disrupted (e.g. feet).

B Prescribe gloves/mittens according to hospital policy.

C Try taping and bandaging tubes for additional security.

D Ask whether a 'special' nurse can be assigned for one-to-one care.

E Tape incontinence pads around Ron's hands to stop him pulling out lines.

29. Ivy has dementia and often screams out all night. Her clinical condition has recently improved and she has become mobile by 'furniture-walking' around the ward. She is violent and abusive when stopped by members of staff.

Rank in order the following actions in response to this situation (1 = Most appropriate; 5 = Least appropriate)

A Try to reason with Ivy, explaining as far as possible that it is unsafe for her to move around the ward.

B Suggest distracting interventions such as playing music.

C Prescribe 'as required' (PRN) sedation.

D Ask whether a 'special' nurse can be assigned for one-to-one care.

E Prescribe sedation when Ivy becomes particularly agitated and endangers herself or others.

30. You are hoping to finish your ward round quickly before meeting your Educational Supervisor an hour later. You see Rose, who is very overweight and disabled with osteoarthritis, sitting in a chair. You are told that she developed severe abdominal pain overnight and so will need to be examined in bed. This will require considerable time as she must be hoisted.

Rank in order the following actions in response to this situation (1 = Most appropriate; 5 = Least appropriate)

A Ask the nursing staff if they can help Rose into bed while you see other patients first.

B Ask Rose whether she would mind lying in bed so that you can examine her thoroughly.

C See Rose later as you are pressed for time.

D See Rose now, but feel her abdomen while she is sitting in the chair instead.

E Go to your meeting with a view to assessing Rose afterwards.

31. Flora is 73 and suffering from hospital-acquired pneumonia. She has been receiving intravenous antibiotics but is no longer confused and is becoming unhappy with your continued attempts at cannulation.

Choose the THREE most appropriate actions to take in this situation

A Tell Flora that she will probably die without intravenous antibiotics.

B Stop the antibiotics and resite the cannula if Flora deteriorates without them.

C Prescribe oral antibiotics, and document clearly that Flora refused cannulation.

D Offer to ask a colleague to try if the next attempt fails.

E Explain carefully why a cannula is necessary.

F Tell Flora that the next attempt will be successful.

G Persist with cannulation attempts as Flora does not have capacity.

H Consider whether antibiotics can be de-escalated to oral equivalents.

32. Randhir is 50 and was admitted under the orthopaedic team with severe back pain. MRI shows only degenerative change. Your consultant says that the patient cannot be kept in hospital 'forever' because of pain and should be discharged with spine surgeon follow-up. The patient and his family do not believe that he can go home because he cannot work and is in severe pain.

Choose the THREE most appropriate actions to take in this situation

A Delete the patient from your list so that he can stay in hospital for a few more days without your consultant knowing.

B Explore Randhir's concerns about going home.

C Promise that you will ensure that the back pain appointment is made within two weeks.

D Tell Randhir that the bed is needed for more urgent cases.

E Carefully explain the nature of mechanical back pain.

F Ensure that the pain team is involved with discharge planning so that appropriate analgesia can be provided in the community.

G Prescribe 'as required' (PRN) oral morphine until the patient is discharged.

H Tell Randhir he needs to learn to accept the pain as there may be nothing that can be done to help.

33. Archie is a 70-year-old man admitted six days previously for an acute coronary syndrome. He has always been polite and pleasant to speak to. However, today he seems unwilling to answer questions directly and you find yourself becoming increasingly annoyed about having to repeat every question to keep him on track.

Choose the THREE most appropriate actions to take in this situation

A Calculate the Abbreviated Mental Test Score (AMTS).

B Tell Archie that you will come back later after you have seen some other patients.

C Document in the notes that Archie is a 'difficult patient'.

D Consider requesting blood tests, urinalysis, and a chest X-ray.

E Just 'eyeball' Archie the following day, rather than seeing him thoroughly on the ward round, as this took a long time the day before.

F Take a full history and examine Archie, even if it is taking longer than usual.

G Ask your consultant if Archie can be discharged soon as he seems to be fed up with being in hospital.

H Move on quickly so that you can continue the ward round.

34. The nurses inform you that one of your patients has died. He had metastatic lung cancer and had been 'do not resuscitate' for weeks. As you arrive at the patient's side room to confirm death, you are aware that the patient's family are all present, having been called by the ward sister.

Choose the THREE most appropriate actions to take in this situation

A Go straight into the room in case another FY1 doctor gets there first.

B Explain why you have arrived and what you intend to do.

C Ask the relatives to leave, as there is a bed crisis and the patient has to be moved to the mortuary.

D Ask everyone present for identification to prove they are close relatives.

E Give the relatives some space and come back later, introducing yourself if they are still there.

F Tell the relatives this is probably what the patient 'would have wanted'.

G Let the relatives choose whether to be in the room or outside while you confirm death.

H Enter the room and commence chest compressions if the patient is pulseless.

35. Mike is an intravenous drug user on the gastroenterology ward with liver failure secondary to hepatitis C. He is currently pre-scribed intravenous methadone, but healthcare staff are struggling to administer this as his veins are overused. He wants to inject his own methadone as he would do at home.

Choose the THREE most appropriate actions to take in this situation

A Discuss with the ward sister as to whether self-injecting is acceptable on the ward.

B Explain that it is never acceptable for patients to administer their own medication.

C Ensure that Mike is familiar with the NHS equipment and safety rules (e.g. sharps disposal).

D Offer Mike oral morphine if he agrees to forego methadone injections.

E Only agree if the procedure is supervised by a member of staff.

F Explain that this is not possible as he is hepatitis C-positive.

G Give Mike a supply of needles and tell him to 'make himself at home'.

H Ask Mike what dose of methadone he usually takes and prescribe this amount.

36. Roger was admitted to your ward following a stroke which has left him with severe weakness down his left side. He was referred to a local rehabilitation hospital three weeks ago and is currently waiting for a bed to become available.

Choose the THREE most appropriate actions to take in this situation

A Ask the ward physiotherapists if they could spend extra time with Roger before a rehabilitation bed becomes available.

B Ensure that daily inflammatory markers are sent in case Roger devel-ops hospital-acquired pneumonia.

C Call the rehabilitation hospital and insist that they find a bed as Roger is at risk of complications (e.g. pressure sores).

D Cross off the routine prescription for daily low-molecular-weight heparin to reduce the number of injections he receives.

E Call the rehabilitation hospital to check Roger's position on the wait-ing list and ensure that they know that he has waited for three weeks.

F Keep Roger informed of his progress up the waiting list.

G Discharge Roger home to bypass the rehabilitation hospital.

H Suggest that Roger's family keep calling the rehabilitation hospital to push his name further up the waiting list.

37. Tom is a bus driver admitted with an epileptiform seizure. Your consultant tells Tom that he must inform the DVLA. Later in the day, Tom says that he cannot tell the DVLA as driving is his job and he has never had a seizure before this one.

Choose the THREE most appropriate actions to take in this situation

A Call his employer anonymously to let them know he is unsafe to drive.

B Tell Tom that you must inform his employer and call them, even if he refuses consent.

C Document clearly any driving advice given to Tom.

D Agree that he is probably not a danger, but tell Tom that he should probably let the DVLA know anyway.

E Call the DVLA anonymously, but keep this from Tom so that your relationship is not disrupted.

F Explain that there is a reasonable possibility of a second seizure.

G Ask Tom's wife to bring in his driving licence and surrender this to the ward sister.

H Explain that you will have to contact the DVLA if he refuses.

38. A staff nurse approaches you with concerns about Mark, a young man with a recently repaired femoral fracture. He insists on wearing his own clothes and will not change into a hospital gown. Friends also bring food in for him (e.g. take-away curries), which upsets other patients.

Choose the THREE most appropriate actions to take in this situation

A Ask Mark to change into a gown because otherwise he is difficult to examine.

B Tell the nurse that there is no good reason why Mark should not wear his own clothes.

C Explain to the nurse that Mark should be able to eat food from outside if he prefers.

D Tell Mark that if he is well enough to eat curry, then he is well enough to be discharged.

E Tell the nurse that the other patients should ask their friends/relatives to bring in food if that is what they want.

F Ask Mark to consider other patients having to eat hospital food before choosing food for his friends to bring.

G Suggest that Mark be swapped with another patient who is currently in a side room with diarrhoea and vomiting.

H Tell the nurse that Sister controls the ward and that she should speak to Mark if there is a problem.

39. You are asked to site a cannula in John, a patient with traumatic brain injury and a permanent Glasgow Coma Scale (GCS) score of 8. He is dehydrated and requires intravenous fluid.

Choose the THREE most appropriate actions to take in this situation

A Explain to the patient what you are going to do.

B Aim blind if you cannot see a target vein, as multiple attempts are unlikely to cause pain.

C Ask a medical student to insert the cannula, as he can try a few times and it will be good practice.

D Defer the job until later, as it is uncomfortable being in the room with someone who is unresponsive.

E Omit washing your hands and cleaning the area, as the patient is unlikely to comment.

F Warn the patient about a 'sharp scratch', as you would for any other.

G Explain to the patient why a cannula is necessary.

H Try to give oral fluid instead to see if this is tolerated.

40. You are on your way to the blood gas analyser with a sample which should not be left out for more than ten minutes. You hear a patient shouting and put your head around the curtain. An elderly patient of the opposite sex you have not met before says they have been sitting on the commode for half an hour and shouting to be helped into bed.

Choose the THREE most appropriate actions to take in this situation

A Tell the patient you are in a hurry.

B Tell the patient you are in a hurry but will come back in ten minutes.

C Offer to help if you can without compromising the sample.

D Say you will let a nurse know that they need help.

E Reassure the patient that someone will probably come to their assistance soon.

F Suggest that the patient pulls the emergency bell to attract the nurses' attention.

G Say you are sorry that they have been there for so long.

H Tell the patient that they should not shout unless there is an emergency as they may alarm other patients.

41. You are the FY1 doctor on a medical ward, and the police telephones the ward to ask you whether a patient will be discharged soon.

Choose the THREE most appropriate actions to take in this situation

A Ask the police to issue a written request for information.

B Refuse.

C Discuss with the patient whether you can disclose the information.

D Refer the request to your consultant.

E Inform the data protection team in your hospital.

F Disclose the information which the police request.

G Ask the ward clerk to speak with the police.

H Offer a vague response so the true details are not disclosed.

42. You realise that you prescribed a potentially dangerous dose of opioids to a patient. One dose was administered by a junior staff nurse.

Choose the THREE most appropriate actions to take in this situation

A Alter the prescription dose that the patient received yesterday.

B Invite the patient and the family to a meeting with your consultant to explain the nature of your error.

C Inform the nurse in charge and complete an incident form.

D Reflect on the error in your e-portfolio.

E Mention the error to your registrar on the ward round later that morning.

F Check on the patient and explain why you are doing so.

G Leave the prescription as it is, as the patient is improving and is highly unlikely to require any further doses.

H Complain to the rota coordinator that your long days are increasing your rate of errors.

43. An elderly patient on the orthogeriatrics ward tells you during your ward round that her husband pushed her over after an argument, which caused her to fall.

Choose the THREE most appropriate actions to take in this situation

A Assess her mental state.

B Try to obtain corroborating witnesses.

C Inform the police.

D Consider involving the safeguarding team.

E Speak with the husband to obtain his perspective.

F Ask the patient what she wants to do.

G Identify individuals with whom the patient can speak comfortably.

H Pass the information on to the patient's daughter.

44. A patient admitted to your ward has been taking a homeopathic remedy for ten years as part of his regular medication. The patient pleads with you to write this up as, without your prescription, the medication will not be administered during his hospital stay.

Choose the THREE most appropriate actions to take in this situation

A Page the on-call pharmacist.

B Explain the discrepancy of this treatment with modern medical principles and how he should abandon this treatment.

C Consult your Trust's prescribing guidelines on alternative medicines.

D Ask the nursing staff to resolve the matter.

E Make a prescribing decision, based on risks and benefits in the way as you would for any other drug.

F Encourage the patient to take his medications surreptitiously, so it does not have to be formally retained and recorded by staff.

G Ask the patient to abandon his homeopathic remedy while an inpatient in case it may interfere with his other medication.

H Offer the patient acupuncture instead.

45. Your registrar tells you that he has begun a sexual relationship with a patient that he met when she was recently admitted under your team.

Rank in order the following actions in response to this situation (1 = Most appropriate; 5 = Least appropriate)

A Ask the patient whether the relationship is consensual.

B Advise the registrar to reconsider the appropriateness of the relationship.

C Inform the GMC.

D If consenting adults, then there is no need to interfere.

E Inform the hospital's safeguarding team.

46. You have failed to catheterize a patient in A&E. You call the urology registrar who is at home, and he asks you to re-attempt the procedure for a fourth time with a different type of catheter. The patient is in considerable pain after the third attempt.

Rank in order the following actions in response to this situation (1 = Most appropriate; 5 = Least appropriate)

A Refuse to re-attempt catheterization without the urology registrar being present.

B Keep trying to catheterize until you are successful, even if the patient refuses.

C Ask the charge nurse to request that the A&E registrar attempts the catheterization.

D Document the urology registrar's request and ask the patient whether he would permit another attempt.

E Prescribe pain relief.

47. Your registrar has asked you to attend A&E to review a child with suspected meningitis. You examine the child and think that a lumbar puncture is required, but have no experience in performing this procedure in children.

Rank in order the following actions in response to this situation (1 = Most appropriate; 5 = Least appropriate)

A Do not proceed, as your inexperience demands supervision.

B You should hide your relative inexperience from the parents and continue until confronted.

C Your registrar has given you permission to independently manage the patient, so you should make the decision alone.

D Explain to the parents your dilemma and offer them the choice.

E Try to speak with the registrar before committing to the lumbar puncture.

ANSWERS

1. D, C, A, B, E

Doctors must work in their patients' interests, while respectfully considering the valuable input of family and friends. The best answer is (D) because it is essential to gain the patient's perspective on each concern in order to address the need for intervention. (C) has the possibility of resolving all of the family's concerns if the patient's cognitive decline is remediable, although it obviously neglects involving the patient in your efforts. You can consider arranging the remaining options in terms of their order of severity and the likelihood of you being able to help. An assessment by the occupational therapist usually identifies and addresses any potential problems with the ability to function at home (A). Financial exploitation lies outside the immediate remit of the clinical team; however, it would be inappropriate for you to ignore any legitimate concerns (B). A local vulnerable adults' nurse or social worker is most qualified to make the appropriate assessments, not a foundation doctor. (E) is a wrong answer as there is no objective evidence of falls in the question, and, in any event, a nursing home would not be the first step to avoiding these in future.

2. A, C, E, B, D

While it is unfortunate to compromise your teaching commitments, hospitals exist for patient well-being first and foremost. There are other ways in which the teaching time can be effectively utilized, and therefore (A) would be the most preferable. A willingness to discontinue is less ideal (C) but is better than the remaining options, as it acknowledges the patient's vulnerability. (E) makes no attempt to even acknowledge the patient's distress and is therefore worse, but has the benefit of being brief and focused on examination which will not necessarily antagonize the patient. In contrast, (B) is an incorrect response; the patient's distress is trivialized into a generic statement about chronic disease, and teaching continues completely unaltered, prolonging the distress for the patient. (D) represents the worst response, as it is likely to worsen the situation by exploring personal family problems in an inappropriate setting with an audience of six medical students.

3. D, C, B, E, A

In any frequently attending patient, it is important to address their background and beliefs to identify any underlying concerns that might be bringing them back. (D) is therefore the best answer, as although the appointment is likely to overrun, it is sometimes necessary to offer additional time, and you may be able to deal with this otherwise complex problem. It is obviously better that you are able to resolve the patient's problems yourself, but if this is not possible, seeking the input of a specialist colleague might be sensible in case you and your colleagues have missed something (C). A trial of non-traditional therapy (B) implies that you have exhausted all appropriate medical therapy (provided of course the diagnosis is correct) and would be a correct option once you had fully explored the patient's psychosocial well-being or sought specialist advice, as described earlier. A fourth colleague at the practice is unlikely to be able to add anything further to the patient's current management and represents a misuse of the practice's resources (E). You should treat each patient independently of other cases; your previous clinical encounters during the day are irrelevant to the care you should provide to this patient. Hence, informing your patient about more 'serious' cases would obviously be the least appropriate option (A).

4. **E, D, A, B, C**

It is your responsibility to work in partnership with your patients and establish and maintain effective relationships with them. (E) is an arbitrary time to spend with the patient, but it does what is necessary to address your consultant's request. (D) is less direct, although a collateral history from the family may shed some light on the patient's concerns. (A) does not really address the problem as no questions are asked and is therefore the least effective 'correct' answer. (B) and (C) are incorrect and represent inappropriate delegations which are unlikely to lead to the desired outcome, with a nurse (B) being only slightly preferable to an HCA (C).

5. **C, E, B, D, A**

In caring for any patient, you should show compassion and develop rapport while maintaining an adequate professional distance. This balance is best made by (C). Nothing in the question invites the response in (E), but it might be helpful to share her personal feelings with someone close whom she trusts. (B) is generally wrong, as it involves disclosing some personal information about yourself, but it may not always be wrong and it could have a positive effect in some patients. (D) is worse as it is dismissive and misses an opportunity to explore an important issue. The worst answer is (A), as it is very unprofessional and irrelevant and may disrupt the relationship with your patient.

6. **A, E, B, C, D**

The patient's wishes must always be followed, even when contrary to their perceived best interests, provided that the patient has capacity to make their own decisions. No diagnosis (e.g. dementia) precludes a patient having capacity, which must be assessed in each case in a time- and decision-specific manner. Therefore, (A) is the only correct answer. (E) is unnecessary, but it is not incorrect or dangerous. (B) implies an incorrect definition of capacity, although the medical notes may be able to shed some light on the patient's previous state, e.g. prior loss of capacity, known dementia, Abbreviated Mental Test Scores on admission, and it is therefore not completely useless. (C) places an unfair burden on the daughter and is inappropriate and incorrect, and it is unhelpful to involve a family member in this way. However, (D) is the worst answer, as it completely ignores the patient's autonomy and is possibly illegal.

7. **C, B, A, E, D**

This question requires you to address patient concerns while also pro-viding reassurance when appropriate. Derek has not offered a suitable indication for a CT scan, but the correct response is to conduct a full assessment, as other decisions cannot be made without this (C). While the patient's risk of developing cancer may be low, you are given no information to be certain of this; it is quite possible the patient may have a cancer syndrome that predisposes him, which makes (B) a less appropriate response. (A) is a fair thing to explain but does not address the patient's anxieties. (E) is obviously incorrect without further clinical information, and not very much better than ordering an inappropriate scan (D).

8. **D, A, E, C, B**

GMC guidance states that drugs should be prescribed to meet the needs of patients and not simply because a patient demands them. (D) rep-resents an honest answer and follows evidence-based/locally agreed guidelines. (A) is an alternative approach and your prerogative, although you would need to have good reasons for doing something different to the consensus of your colleagues. (E) is likely to be unhelpful, as it simply defers the decision-making to a colleague, although it is not incorrect. (C) might be necessary if you wanted funding for a drug, but it is not necessary to prescribe it. (B) is the only explicitly wrong answer, as it may be unsafe for the patient to purchase medication from an unlicensed supplier.

9. **A, D, C, E, B**

It is necessary to foster a professional relationship with every patient by establishing rapport and understanding their concerns, and this may lead to identifying why the patient is refusing the procedure and possibly how to overcome this (A). (D) is not incorrect and might allow the patient's concerns about the procedure to be answered, albeit indirectly, but is less effective than (A). (C) is also not incorrect but is unlikely to achieve a resolution, and is less appropriate than exploring the patient's concerns directly with the patient. (B) and (E) are clearly incorrect answers and it is difficult to decide which is worst. It is never appropriate to insist on a patient having a treatment, unless they do not have capacity and a 'best interests' decision has been made (E); instead the pros and cons of each option should be discussed with the patient. This option is probably not the very worst action, as it stops short of actually going ahead with the procedure without the patient's consent (i.e. battery). (B) is probably marginally worse than (E), as it is completely inappropriate for the patient and breaches the confidentiality of another patient at the same time.

10. **D, C, B, A, E**

Your first duty should be towards your patient; *Good Medical Practice* also reminds us to work with colleagues effectively to best serve patients' interests. In this instance, you should aim to get the patient referred as early as possible, even if this means involving the consultant. Clearly, speaking to the SHO directly is better than involving the consultant if this can be avoided, hence (D) is better than (C). Involving the nurses (B) requires that they become involved in a task they are not supposed to do, and this is therefore less preferential. However, it is better than (A) which leaves the task (and therefore the patient) until the end of the day. (E) is clearly the worst, as it leaves the patient in pain for the longest duration.

11. **A, D, E**

Confidentiality is central to the trust between patients and doctors. The disclosure of information in the interest of public safety is a complex issue, requiring a balanced and thoughtful clinical judgement in discussion with the patient. In this scenario, it is recommended to complete a sexual diseases screening to rule out common or serious infections (D), although no disease *must* be tested for (C). It would be unfair to defer phlebotomy to another healthcare professional (H) simply because you are worried. At this stage, it is not appropriate to consider disclosure of the patient's sexual encounter to her partner or GP (B) (G), although she might be encouraged to share this information herself (A). Such clinical encounters provide the opportunity to promote safe sexual practices (E), but personal opinions about patients' sexual practices should remain private (F).

12. **D, F, H**

This common scenario represents many priorities which must be balanced, the most important of which is patient care. Ward telephones should be answered promptly, even if it is not an individual's direct responsibility because they carry a bleep. The staff nurse may be more persuaded to help if you have their prior agreement (D). It might just be easier to answer the phone quickly, work out what the call is about, and move on (F). You may have unrealistically expected to see a patient within ten minutes, as well as making it to lunch on time. It is often useful to lead by example, in which case simply expecting others to act may be unhelpful (A) (B) (C). Only if the difficulty persists and/or this is a ward that you are likely to visit again should you need to find out the policy on answering telephones (G). Giving the handset directly to the staff nurse (E) would be bad manners and unlikely to provoke a positive response, particularly as you do not know the urgency of the task he is currently managing. Ultimately the call might be important and should be answered, and although (H) is imposing and it might be difficult to interrupt others in the middle of their own jobs, it is the least worst of the remaining options after (D) and (F).

13. **A, B, D, C, E**

You must ensure patient safety by raising your concerns, and there is a fairly clear order of escalation. In this scenario, (A) is better than (B), as it is more appropriate to formally raise the issue again with the consultant and reiterate your concerns with specific examples of what you believe has been done incorrectly. It is possible that your assessment is inaccurate or disproportionate, and discussion with a senior colleague may be helpful in this respect. In any event, if the evidence is unequivocal, the registrar will benefit from the input of a senior clinician. Informing the Clinical Director (D) represents a greater escalation than your Educational Supervisor (who is another consultant typically responsible for fewer staff than the Clinical Director). It may eventually be appropriate to inform the Clinical Director, although you should escalate stepwise through the local hierarchy. It would be ideal to approach the registrar himself; however, offering him teaching is unlikely to be constructive and, in this case, would not be appropriate (C). If, however, the option was to approach the registrar and to discuss your concerns further with him, this would have been the best option. (E) is the worst option, as it amounts to gossiping and will not lead to the problem being resolved.

14. B, C, D

Good Medical Practice reminds us to listen to patients and to spend time with relatives and respond to their concerns and preferences. In this scenario, where the child does not speak English, you should try to understand the family's particular health beliefs before communicating via them with Lenka to identify her concerns (C) (D). The family may be unsettled by conditions on the ward, but the neighbouring patient is unlikely to pose a risk to Lenka (B) and any patients who are at risk of transmitting infectious diseases would already be isolated. Therefore, it is unnecessary and an inappropriate use of resources to isolate Lenka or the neighbouring patient (A) (E), or to provide face masks (F) (H). Since you have begun to speak to the patient's family and can respond to their concerns, it would be unfair to refer them to the ward nurse (G).

15. E, B, C, A, D

The GMC requires doctors to treat patients fairly and not to discriminate unfairly between them. In this instance, your colleague may be abusing his position to gain preferential treatment, but it is possible that his professional insight has raised a concern which *should* expedite his father's care. For this reason, (E) is the best option.

(B) and (C) are difficult to choose between and will depend on several factors not discussed, e.g. the department or other patients. It is important to weight fairness against working with colleagues, and your registrar may be able to offer additional insight and help triage the patients waiting to be clerked (however, this requires involving a likely very busy registrar with a query that is questionable at best). On balance, most doctors would say it is better to decline your former colleague's request if there is no good reason. (A) is unfair and excessive, while (D) is all of these explanations given *and* dangerous, and is clearly the worst option.

16. E, B, C, A, D

Failing to give Lucy her medications could put her at unacceptable risk. There is a suggestion that the nurse has neglected an important duty, and the ward sister should be requested to investigate the matter further, hence (E) is the best option. (C) also raises the concern with nursing staff, but only with the nurse involved, and would address the matter if the problem was patient compliance, but not if there was an issue with the nurse's dispensing of medication. (B) does not resolve the situation immediately but goes about initiating the same processes that the ward sister would begin in (E); therefore, (B) can be justified as being better than (C). (A) is incorrect without further corroboration/information. (D) does not adequately address the failure by the nurse or the patient's non-compliance for the future and is potentially dangerous, introducing unnecessary risk to the patient.

17. E, D, B, C, A

It is essential that there is adequate communication between the patient and the clinical team. The revelation that Mr Stevenson and his family do not know about the DNACPR order warrants a discussion with your senior, but the scenario does not imply any immediate imminent danger, hence this is not *immediately* necessary. (E) would therefore be preferable to (D), as it allows you to establish what the patient has already discussed (perhaps in private, away from his family) and discuss the matter with your seniors further if necessary. (B) is probably not a discussion that should be undertaken by an FY1 doctor, particularly if the issue had never been raised before. (C) is the first wrong answer, as you cannot apologize for colleagues and do not know what he was previously told and why. (A) is the worst answer, as you do not know why the DNACPR was put in place, or by whom, and you are not in a good position to make DNACPR decisions.

18. C, D, B, E, A

Although Clara's description may represent reasonable chastisement, the issue should be explored as it might indicate non-accidental injury. (C) is the best option, as it ensures the comments have been recorded and allows further detail to be established which may clarify what she means, or else highlight further concerns which can then be shared with an appropriate senior colleague. Accurate contemporaneous documentation is always key, and such cases might be followed up by external agencies and your information relied upon in court. (D) is not ideal and risks antagonizing the mother if she probes further, but it is important to assess the patient, and in this instance your honesty would not be unacceptable. (B) would generally be considered incorrect for an FY1 doctor to undertake independently and is therefore worse. (E) is a disproportionate and excessive response that is by no means justified at this stage, although it is marginally better than (A) which completely ignores the potential seriousness of Clara's disclosure.

19. D, B, A, C, E

Although confidentiality is necessary to maintain patient trust in doctors, it may be breached to protect others from serious harm. Terence has a legal duty to inform the DVLA, which is likely to ask him to surrender his licence. The best answer would be to encourage the patient to disclose his disability and, failing this, to do so yourself. (D) represents the safest option available and is therefore the best option. The remaining options are generally inappropriate. (B) at least informs another colleague that there is an issue, who could follow the issue up further. (A) is worse, as the wife might not be trusted, given her conflict of interest, and this represents an unfair burden as she might not be able to control her husband, although there is a possibility she would be able to prevent him from driving. (C) is tantamount to doing nothing and adds nothing on top of a verbal reassurance. (E) is obviously wrong and neglects a duty to protect public safety.

20. A, D, C, B, E

It is often necessary to strike a careful balance between reassurance and fostering a realistic outlook that does not compromise the patient's faith in the profession. At this stage, you cannot fully reassure the patient and instead must be honest about her situation (A). (D) is the next best answer; although it would be odd and unlikely to help the patient, it is a neutral statement. (C) is worse, as it burdens your seniors unnecessarily, particularly since the patient has not asked for any specific information. It is difficult to discriminate between the last two options. (B) is incorrect, and (E) is ambiguous, confusing, and unfair to the patient. The implication of a poor outcome without explicitly stating so is perhaps worse than a falsely reassuring comment made in passing.

21. C, B, A, D, E

All healthcare professionals should respect patient autonomy and empower patients as far as possible. It is better to speak to the nurses before promising anything directly to the patient; therefore, (C) is a better option than (B). It is unfair not to pass on the patient's (reasonable) request to the nursing staff; therefore, the remaining answers are incorrect. (A) is probably the better of those remaining, as it might be good for the patient's morale. (D) is less effective than (A), as it fails to address the problem and represents a less positive, more neutral statement. (E) has the same failings as (D), possibly carrying a more negative undertone, but more importantly is factually incorrect.

22. A, B, C, D, E

You should only offer invasive treatment if it is in the patient's interest and you have consent. (A) is the most patient-focused response and will help guide you to the correct management for the patient. (B) is less effective, as it fails to establish a history and the patient's perspective about his symptoms, although he is involved in the decision-making and the options offered are less invasive. (C) is likely to be unnecessary in this case, but it is not harmful, although it may delay a speedier resolution which could be achieved without having to involve another specialist team. (D) is less effective than (C), as it is mildly harmful to insert a catheter, but it is done correctly by explaining the procedure and obtaining consent. For this reason, (D) is better than (E), as the consent obtained with this option (E) is somewhat dubious.

23. A, C, D, E, B

You should take steps to protect patient dignity whenever possible. (A) is the most immediate way to achieve this. (C) is a less immediate action but still offers a sensible approach. (D) is unprofessional, as it undermines your nursing colleague, but it is not completely incorrect, as the underlying issue is still addressed. For this reason, (D) is better than (E), as ignoring the issue is slightly worse. Patient choice is important, but other patients and visitors to the ward need to be considered as well, and it would be considered poor judgement to attempt to address the issue only to go on and leave the curtains open (B).

24. A, E, D, B, C

It is important that patients have an opportunity to ask questions, particularly about such an important issue. In this case, indicating to the patient that you will come back addresses the main issue raised in the question, without disrupting the ward round, and is the best answer (A). This is preferable to simply going back later (E), as it will reassure the patient immediately to know there will be an additional opportunity to ask further questions, although (E) does still deal with the underlying issue. (D) is good for the patient but inevitably disrupts the ward round and is therefore less preferable. (B) is worse than (D), as it is unprofessional and causes maximum disruption to the rest of the ward round. (B) and (C) are difficult to discriminate, and arguments can be made for both being the worst answer. One can argue that (B) carries a greater risk of jeopardizing your professional relationship with the consultant by insisting on his cooperation in front of the patient, compared to falsely promising a meeting with the consultant (C) (a meeting that you might be able to effectively negotiate more politely than is implied in option (B)). They are both unprofessional, but for the patient, (C) is worse as you cannot guarantee that the consultant will return, and this risks leaving the patient's questions entirely unanswered.

25. B, C, D, E, A

You should take action as necessary to protect patient dignity. In this case, (B) is the most helpful and polite response. (C) is a reasonable action, but it would be preferable to speak to him as in (B) first. It would be better to deal with the patient's immediate (and easily correctable, be it non-life-threatening) problem yourself and avoid delay, rather than seeking a nurse (D). The two remaining options are incorrect, with (A) being impolite and (E) being even more unkind by blaming the patient for a genuine mistake.

26. D, E, C, B, A

Mittens risk causing patients significant distress and should only be used in limited circumstances. Most Trusts have strict criteria and rules for their use, for example the patient should either consent or lack capacity, and had previously pulled out lines and tubes, and alternative strategies have been unsuccessful. Hence (D) is the correct answer. The hostile family members are likely to dissuade you from the use of mittens, but cooperation is not a requirement, and therefore (E) is an appropriate (albeit less ideal) response. (C) represents a partial requirement, while (B) is even less appropriate as it represents less fulfilment of the required conditions for using mittens. (A) is not really necessary, even for the use of mittens, and is therefore the worst answer.

27. **B, D, A, C, E**

(B) is the best answer, as it is most likely to resolve the problem and offers appropriate counselling to the patient. It is obviously preferable to resolve the problem with the patient and obtain his consent for sharing information with the HPA, but telling the patient that you will be informing them is a fair and reasonable response (D). However, (D) is not as effective as (B), as the immediate risk to other people is minimized by explaining the seriousness of the condition and why the restrictions are being imposed on him. While you should generally explore all reasons for non-compliance (as patients might be amenable to persuasion), you are unlikely to impart the essential information that he has a communicable disease which might currently risk others, and that this should be reported to the HPA (A). (C) is incorrect, as the HPA must be informed, while (E) is both incorrect and represents a failure to treat the patient, putting him and others at considerable risk from untreated tuberculosis.

28. **C, A, D, B, E**

Ron may cause himself considerable harm by inadvertently pulling out lines and tubes. You should ensure Ron's safety using the minimum amount of restrictions. The order of answers suggested here is an appropriate order of escalation, and so almost by definition the next stage is 'less appropriate' than the one before. Bandages (C) are less invasive than resiting cannulae (A), while specialist one-to-one nursing (D) might be able to obviate the more restrictive option which is often a last resort—mittens (B). Mittens should only be used as a last resort when other strategies have failed and according to Trust policy. Taping pads to Ron's hands would be undignified and uncomfortable, and may worsen his agitation (E). If hands must be constrained, specially designed mittens should be used according to policy.

29. **A, B, D, E, C**

The correct order of answers here represents a clear order of escalation, beginning with the more conservative least invasive methods first. Sedation should only be prescribed when it is in your patient's interests. The interests of colleagues and other patients are secondary in this case. Although Ivy has dementia, attempts should be made to explain to her that she is unsafe to mobilize (A). Other alternatives to sedation can then be explored, such as distraction (B). One-to-one nursing might be required and may be successful, but it is obviously resource-intensive and this needs to be considered (D). Sedation may be considered when Ivy becomes particularly agitated and a risk to herself (E), although prescribing the medication when necessary would be favoured over 'PRN' sedation (C) to avoid the patient being oversedated by nursing staff.

30. B, A, D, E, C

Patient care must be prioritized, even above educational commitments. The concern is that Rose has a possible acute abdomen and therefore needs to be examined properly. The best answer is (B) which informs her about your intentions and is clearly a better use of resources than (A). Both options are, however, preferable to conducting an inadequate examination of a patient who has potentially become very unwell (D). (E) and (C) are the worst answers, as they both neglect any assessment of Rose. (E) is only marginally better, as you are at least making an effort to attend your meeting.

31. D, E, H

Competent adults can refuse any treatment, including cannulation. However, you have a duty to ensure that they understand the reason it is necessary and the likely consequences of refusal (E). This might be an appropriate time to consider converting to oral antibiotics (H) or a compromise might be necessary, such as offering to seek help from a colleague after another attempt (D). You should not accept Flora's refusal of further attempts without clear discussion of the need for intravenous antibiotics (C). This discussion should be realistic and not calculated to coerce the patient (A). You cannot guarantee that the next attempt will be successful (F) and there is no reason to think that Flora does not have capacity (G). Antibiotics should not be stopped in their entirety (B) simply because Flora is declining cannulation—oral equivalents may confer some benefit.

32. B, E, F

Compromise is always preferable and can only be achieved by understanding Randhir's concerns (B) and clarifying any misunderstandings (E). Regardless of conflict persisting, the discharge should be managed like any other with effective analgesia and follow-up (F). You should not make unhelpful statements, for example that nothing can be done to help (H) or that the bed is needed for 'more urgent' cases (D).

You should never mislead your consultant over which patients are under their care (A). It is unlikely that you can guarantee the timescale on which outpatient appointments are made (C). Regular strong opiate analgesia may be unhelpful if this cannot be continued in the community (G). This strategy should only be considered on specialist advice.

33. A, D, F

It is important not to let feelings cloud your professional judgement. The concern here is that Archie has become confused, which might be apparent objectively on calculating his AMTS (A). Otherwise unexplained personality changes warrant a full history, examination (F), and septic screen (D).

Your personal feelings should not cause you to move on prematurely (B) (H) or avoid seeing Archie (E) the following day. Documenting that Archie is a 'difficult patient' (C) adds little to his care. Conspiring to promote an early discharge is also unhelpful if Archie's personality change is the result of a pathological event (G).

34. B, E, G

Although formal confirmation of death should be done promptly, other considerations may be prioritized. The relatives may appreciate some time with the patient, after which you should introduce yourself (E) and explain what the process involves (B). You should let the relatives choose whether to vacate the room (G), as some aspects (e.g. checking for pupillary reflexes) might distress them.

There is no need to ask for identification (D), make trite comments which may cause offence (F), or commence chest compressions (H) if there is a valid 'do not resuscitate' instruction. Financial (A) and bed management considerations (C) have no place at this time.

35. A, C, E

Any decisions about behaviour on the ward should be made in collaboration with the nursing staff (A). If it is agreed that Mike can administer his own methadone, he must be familiar with the equipment and safety requirements (C), and supervised (E) to ensure that sharps are appropriately discarded.

It would be inadvisable to alter Mike's regimen (D) without specialist advice or to give him needles (G) without addressing the issues described previously. Patients are often allowed to administer their own medication (B) (e.g. self-injecting insulin) when this is agreed with the nursing staff.

Hepatitis C emphasizes the importance of disposing of sharps safely but does not alter whether the process of self-injecting is permissible (F). Doctors should not usually accept the dose of methadone that someone who is drug-dependent has said they are usually prescribed (H). Independent verification is necessary (e.g. from a GP or pharmacy).

36. A, E, F

Doctors must advocate appropriately for their patients. If the wait is unusual, you should contact the rehabilitation hospital to check that Roger has not been missed (E). You should keep Roger informed (F) and ask the ward physiotherapists to do their best to mitigate the disadvantage of remaining in an acute hospital bed (A).

However, you should be sensitive to the resource allocations of other healthcare providers. Asking Roger's family to campaign (H) at the expense of other patients or insisting that the rehabilitation hospital find a bed (C) may be unhelpful. Daily inflammatory markers are inappropriate in a 'well' patient (B), but low-molecular-weight heparin should probably continue as his mobility is impaired (D). Discharge would only be appropriate if the multi-disciplinary team agree that Roger has returned to baseline and no longer requires prolonged rehabilitation (G),

37. C, F, H

Tom has a legal duty to inform the DVLA. Although this legal duty does not extend to doctors, you have a professional duty to balance the need for confidentiality against harm occurring to others. Therefore, you cannot conspire with Tom to keep his driving secret (D).

You should ensure that Tom is fully informed about the risk of a second seizure (F) and that this advice is documented carefully (C). Your professional duty probably requires informing the DVLA if Tom refuses (H), but this should be made clear to him (E). Although it could be justifiable to inform Tom's employer, this is a more radical step and probably unnecessary if the DVLA is notified (B) (A). The hospital has no role to play in confiscating Tom's driving licence (G).

38. B, C, F

There is no obvious reason why Mark should wear a hospital gown (B) (A) and he certainly cannot be forced to wear one. Similarly, there is no clinical reason why Mark should be confined to hospital food (C). However, if this is having a negative impact on other patients, it may be worth bringing this to Mark's attention (F). Although the ward sister might want to talk to Mark, there is no reason why you should not do so (H).

It cannot be assumed that all patients have people willing to bring them food (E), and neither does it follow that Mark must be fit enough for discharge (D). Moving Mark to a side room is a possibility, but only if one is available. He should certainly not be swapped for a patient isolated for clinical reasons (e.g. diarrhoea and vomiting) (G).

39. A, F, G

Although the patient has a GCS of 8, it is impossible to know to what extent he is aware of his surroundings. Therefore, you should assume that he can hear and understand. You should explain the procedure fully (A) (G) and give warnings when appropriate (F).

You should not treat John differently because he is unresponsive, for example by careless attempts at cannulation (B), omission of important steps (E), or delegating the task inappropriately (C). John is a vulnerable patient as he cannot advocate for himself, and so his care should not be deferred until later (D). Giving oral fluid to an unresponsive patient is likely to result in aspiration (H).

40. C, D, G

In this scenario, you must balance the dignity and comfort of one patient against the need to take a second blood sample from another. You should certainly help the patient on the commode if you are able to (C) or ask a nurse to do so (D). Clearly, it is not appropriate for a patient to be left on the commode shouting, and it is likely the nurses are occupied elsewhere. You could apologize for this without the need to assign blame (G). Clearly, reprimanding the patient for shouting is not helpful (H). Letting the patient know that you are in a hurry is only helpful if it precedes your assurance that someone else will help shortly (A) (B). A vague reassurance that 'someone' will 'probably' help soon is unhelpful (E). The patient should not be encouraged to abuse their emergency bell (F).

41. A, C, D

The key to this question is not to disclose the patient's information without their consent (C), irrespective of who is asking. There are exceptions to this (e.g. some serious crimes and overriding public interest), but there is no evidence of such circumstances in the stem. In asking the police to direct their request to your consultant (D), or state it in writing (A), you will have provided an opportunity to consult the patient and anyone else that might need to advise you, should the patient withhold their consent. This might seem unnecessarily unhelpful, but the patient's confidentiality is—in general terms—prioritized above the needs of the police to discharge their obligations.

Options that are deliberately unclear (H), needlessly directing the police to the different departments (E), or diverting them to inappropriate colleagues (G) are all unhelpful.

42. C, D, F

It may be necessary to escalate the issue further if a serious untoward incident had occurred, but it is not suggested by the scenario (B) (E) (H). However, given this was a prescription-related error, it would be appropriate to reflect on your mistake (D), as well as informing the nursing hierarchy so that they could feed back to the nurse who administered the incorrect dose (C). You should certainly check that the patient did not come to any harm and the duty of candour ideally requires that you inform the patient about the error (F).

It would clearly be dangerous to leave the prescription in place (G) or alter the dose of a prescription that has already been administered (A).

43. A, D, F

The most overriding responsibility in this scenario is to promote the safety of a potentially vulnerable adult. When a disclosure is made about domestic violence, you should usually be guided by the patient as to how they would like to proceed (F). Although it might well end up involving the police, this would usually require the patient to want to pursue this course of action (C). However, you will want to have a low threshold for sharing information with the local safeguarding team who could advise you further (D).

It is worth being aware that older adults on surgical wards are vulnerable to cognitive impairment (delirium and/or dementia) that will sometimes manifest as false accusations. It is therefore worth making some assessment as to whether this is an issue for the current patient (A). That said, you will clearly need to take the allegation seriously and beware that domestic violence and cognitive impairment can easily coexist.

It is clearly not your role to investigate further by speaking to the husband (E), potential witnesses (B), or other relatives (H).

44. **A, C, E**

You should treat homeopathic drugs in this scenario like any other medication. If the patient felt strongly about taking their medication, it would be reasonable to continue it, along with other regular drugs, unless you had a reason to think it risked harm and so could not take responsibility for the prescription (E). You might want to speak with the pharmacist or consult your local guidelines, particularly if your patient needs repeat dispensing of medication that they do not have with them (A) (E). Surreptitious dosing of medications is not to be encouraged (F), and trying to influence the patient's long-standing commitment to alternative medicines seems unlikely to be effective (B) (G) (H). Passing the problem on to the nursing staff (D) is unlikely to solve the issue or endear you to your colleagues.

45. **B, E, A, C, D**

It is never appropriate to engage in a personal relationship with patients and the sooner this situation can be resolved the better, hence (B) being the best option and (D) the worst. Option (E) could be relevant if there was an ongoing safeguarding issue, which arguably is not the case from the information provided in the stem and may be marginally more relevant in certain circumstances. It is clearly not your role to investigate further (A), and referral to the GMC would likely be an over-reaction at this stage, particularly as the patient does not appear to be under the care of your team any longer (C). There may well be disciplinary implications for the registrar, depending on the circumstances, e.g. when the relationship developed.

46. **D, E, C, A, B**

It is clearly important to obtain consent for any procedure, but a fourth attempt under such circumstances may require additional explanation. Advice from specialists should be documented contemporaneously (D). It is important to ensure the patient has adequate pain relief (E), although this follows (D) as it does not solve the immediate issue at hand. Although it might be appropriate to seek help from a more experienced doctor, it would be courteous to do this directly, rather than indirectly through a third party (C). If the urologist has advised a further attempt and the patient agrees, it would be unhelpful to refuse to continue (A). It would be unethical and unlawful to continue attempts at catherization without the patient's consent (B).

47. **E, A, C, B, D**

Option (E) offers the opportunity to consult with a senior colleague and assess whether it would be appropriate for you to proceed with this urgent investigation. You should not perform procedures unsupervised, unless you are competent to do so, but (A) comes after (E) as the latter at least suggests a way of getting the procedure done.

Option (C) is wrong as it suggests that you cannot seek assistance. This is, however, preferable to (B), which suggests an unsafe course of action (performing a procedure unsupervised when you are not competent to do so) and dishonesty. (D) is—just about—worse than (B) as it risks confusing the parents and undermining their confidence in doctors, and also suggests willingness to perform the procedure unsupervised.

Working effectively as part of a team

Introduction

Teamworking is an inevitable part of working within a complex multi-disciplinary environment. Thankfully, most interactions with other members of the healthcare team will be positive and constructive. Unfortunately, such happy circumstances do not make for particularly interesting SJT scenarios. The following section is therefore full of colleagues that are angry, rude, dishonest, unprofessional, and even intoxicated. In *Raising and Acting on Concerns About Patient Safety* (2012), the General Medical Council (GMC) states that 'all doctors have a duty to raise concerns where they believe that patient safety or care is being compromised by the practice of colleagues or the systems, policies and procedures in the organizations in which they work'. The GMC proposes taking the following steps in sequence when you develop serious concerns about a colleague:

- Raise the concern with 'your manager or an appropriate officer of the organisation ... such as the consultant in charge of the team, the clinical or medical director'. Alternatively, a foundation doctor may raise their concern with an appropriate person responsible for training such as their Foundation Programme Director.

- Raise the concern with a regulator (such as the GMC), professional body (such as the British Medical Association), or charity (such as Public Concern at Work). This step should be taken if you have exhausted options for raising the concern internally and there is an 'immediate serious risk to patients, and a regulator or other external body has responsibility to act or intervene'.

- Raise the concern publicly. This step should be taken when you have exhausted options for raising the concern internally and have 'good reason to believe that patients are still at risk of harm'. Your usual duty is to avoid breaching patient confidentiality. This is a highly unusual and significant step to take and is unlikely to be appropriate without first having taken advice from an appropriate organization such as the GMC, BMA, or Public Concern at Work.

The questions within this section highlight your ability and willingness to work with team members. You will need to work collaboratively and respectfully within a multi-disciplinary team, as well as provide advice and support to colleagues. A willingness to take on more responsibility must always be balanced by an openness to share your workload when necessary.

You should always favour a collaborative approach when answering SJT questions, and part of this domain requires an understanding of your role and the role of others. Recognizing skills and qualities allows you to adapt and demonstrate leadership by utilizing the skills of appropriate individuals to achieve specific goals.

- Different individuals and professions will bring unique perspectives which might result in conflict. Understand what each person is trying to achieve, and remember that you all share the goal of making patients better.

- Respect the fact that other team members have multiple demands on their time. Only they can truly know the extent of their workload.

- Equally, remember that you are an autonomous professional as well with your own responsibilities, e.g. not to be pressured into doing anything that you believe risks harming a patient.

- Try to resolve conflict with the individuals concerned before escalating issues unnecessarily. When an issue arises with a non-doctor, this might best be resolved using their own hierarchy. The nursing staff, including healthcare assistants (HCAs), are supervised by a Ward Sister or Ward Manager who will often answer to a Matron.

- When conflict arises with experienced staff about a *medical* decision, the best answer is often to involve someone from your own hierarchy, i.e. a more senior doctor. Your consultant is ultimately responsible for every patient under his or her care.

References and further reading

Academy of Medical Royal Colleges (2010). *Medical Leadership Competency Framework*. https://www.leadershipacademy.nhs.uk/wp-content/uploads/2012/11/NHSLeadership-Leadership-Framework-Medical-Leadership-Competency-Framework-3rd-ed.pdf

General Medical Council (2012). *Leadership and Management For All Doctors*. http://www.gmc-uk.org/Leadership_and_management_for_all_doctors___English_1015.pdf_48903400.pdf

QUESTIONS

1. A porter tells you that he has seen an HCA take something from a patient's personal belongings.

Rank in order the following actions in response to this situation (1 = Most appropriate; 5 = Least appropriate)

A Ask the HCA to open her locker and empty her pockets.

B Establish exactly what the porter has seen, and confirm with the patient that they have something missing before informing the Ward Sister.

C Call the police.

D Ask the porter to find out more by speaking to the patient and HCA.

E Report the incident to your consultant.

2. You are on a renal medicine ward round and notice your consultant loses his balance but quickly corrects himself. You find his behaviour slightly unusual and can smell alcohol on his breath. Although the decisions he is making appear appropriate, you wonder if he has been drinking alcohol earlier in the day.

Rank in order the following actions in response to this situation (1 = Most appropriate; 5 = Least appropriate)

A Ask the consultant whether he has been drinking alcohol.

B Speak to the consultant's secretary about his behaviour.

C Discuss your concerns with your registrar, and ask whether he feels that the consultant is acting out of character.

D Inform the Clinical Director.

E Speak with the consultant, and share your concerns about what you think you have seen recently.

3. You have asked a nurse to administer a heparin infusion. On returning to the ward three hours later, you find that the infusion has still not been given as the nurse has been busy with other tasks.

Rank in order the following actions in response to this situation (1 = Most appropriate; 5 = Least appropriate)

A Explain the urgency of giving the heparin, and ask her to prepare the infusion straightaway.

B Avoid antagonizing the nurse by leaving her to complete her jobs.

C Speak to the nurse in charge about the delay.

D Confront the nurse on the ward, and insist that she prepares the infusion straightaway.

E Go to the preparation room, and prepare the heparin infusion yourself.

4. It is your first day on the neurology ward, and all junior doctors are changing jobs. You are asked by the ward clerk to complete a discharge summary for a patient who was discharged last week, including arrangements for follow-up.

Rank in order the following actions in response to this situation (1 = Most appropriate; 5 = Least appropriate)

A Refuse and ask the ward clerk to find the foundation doctor who was looking after the patient.

B Ask the new SHO to try to complete it.

C Attempt to complete the discharge summary, and try to find the consultant and ask them about follow-up arrangements.

D Write a letter to the previous junior doctor for the neurology ward, and ask them to complete the discharge summary for their patient.

E Complete the discharge summary to the best of your ability, and arrange routine clinic follow-up in six weeks.

5. A patient approaches you to say that she overheard your registrar swearing repeatedly when he was at the nursing station. She does not wish to make a formal complaint at the moment but suggests that you do something about his language.

Rank in order the following actions in response to this situation (1 = Most appropriate; 5 = Least appropriate)

A Raise the concern privately with your registrar.

B Inform PALS.

C Apologize to the patient, and assure her that you will speak to the doctor involved.

D Establish what exactly was said and when.

E Explain that the registrar is 'only human' and that she should not listen to conversations at the nursing station as they might be confidential.

6. You are working with Dr Green, a GP, about whom you are concerned because he never seems to examine his patients. He appears willing to refer some patients and send others home without as much as a basic physical examination. However, he is well liked by his patients and colleagues, and he has never been subject to a complaint or any disciplinary action.

Choose the THREE most appropriate actions to take in this situation

A You have no substantial proof of malpractice and therefore cannot report your concerns at the moment.

B The collective support of Dr Green at the practice should dissuade you from making a complaint.

C Telephone the GMC to raise your concerns with them.

D Ask the GP about his decisions not to examine patients.

E Attempt to discuss the issue privately with other colleagues at the practice.

F Inform the Primary Care Trust.

G Contact your Educational Supervisor.

H Inform the British Medical Association.

7. Your registrar inadvertently prescribes a ten-times dose of methotrexate which you spot before the first dose is given. The registrar breathes a sigh of relief that the error was spotted and tells you both he and the patient had a 'lucky escape'.

Rank in order the following actions in response to this situation (1 = Most appropriate; 5 = Least appropriate)

A Agree that you are lucky as well, as you would have to complete a long clinical incident form if it had been administered.

B Raise the issue with the nursing staff, so that they are aware of common mistakes to look out for.

C Mention the prescribing error to the lead pharmacist.

D Raise the issue with your consultant at the next ward round.

E Complete a formal incident report.

8. At a multi-disciplinary team meeting, a nurse expresses concern about a patient's ability to mobilize safely at home. The occupational therapy team disagrees, and an argument ensues. Five minutes later, they are continuing to argue, and no progress has been made.

Rank in order the following actions in response to this situation (1 = Most appropriate; 5 = Least appropriate)

A Move the agenda on to the next patient, and return to the controversial case at the end.

B Ask the nurse to elaborate on her concerns.

C Ask the occupational therapist to leave the meeting.

D Invite the social worker to share her opinion.

E Do not become involved.

9. You are an FY1 doctor in orthopaedics. You have found the physiotherapist to be particularly challenging to work with. She frequently ignores the post-operative plan for mobilizing patients and seems to actively discourage patients being discharged home. Your registrar says that the physiotherapist is 'obstructive'.

Rank in order the following actions in response to this situation (1 = Most appropriate; 5 = Least appropriate)

A Speak to the other members of the multi-disciplinary team prior to weekly meetings to establish the discharge plan.

B Ask for the physiotherapist to be replaced.

C Invite the physiotherapist to join your consultant ward round, so that discharge arrangements can be made face-to-face.

D Ask an impartial senior colleague for advice.

E Follow the physiotherapist's advice, as she is ultimately responsible for the patient's safe mobilization.

10. You have been working as the FY1 doctor in the Medical Assessment Unit for two months. On many occasions during the rushed morning handover, you have found that tasks are not appropriately transferred from the night doctors to the morning team. The ethos is focused on handing over quickly, so that the night team can get home to sleep.

Rank in order the following actions in response to this situation (1 = Most appropriate; 5 = Least appropriate)

A Ensure that your own handover is effective.

B Arrange a meeting with your colleagues to explain your concerns.

C File incident reports for each individual whom you believe to be failing in their responsibilities.

D Only comment if urgent tasks are not handed over, as it is not worth making a fuss over routine jobs.

E Inform the consultant in charge that handover arrangements are inadequate.

11. Frances, an FY1 colleague, confides in you that she was recently diagnosed with thyroid cancer. She does not appear to be symptomatic and is scheduled to undergo a biopsy and surgical treatment at another hospital in a month's time. Although she is not as spritely as usual, you have not noticed any change in her performance.

Rank in order the following actions in response to this situation (1 = Most appropriate; 5 = Least appropriate)

A Suggest that she refers herself for counselling via Occupational Health.

B Advise Frances to inform her Educational Supervisor.

C Inform your consultant immediately.

D Gently explore how she is feeling about the diagnosis.

E Keep an eye on Frances at work, but do not say anything to anyone else.

12. Rachel, a fellow FY1 doctor, is a budding surgeon and frequently abandons the ward so that she can assist in theatre. Except for the morning ward round, you have not seen Rachel on the ward for at least five weeks. Your consultant appears content with this arrangement as long as the tasks are completed, and you do not have a particular interest in surgery.

Rank in order the following actions in response to this situation (1 = Most appropriate; 5 = Least appropriate)

A Do nothing as you enjoy the ward and Rachel clearly wants to be in theatre.

B Speak to Rachel and insist that she spends more time on the ward.

C Go to theatre and leave any ward jobs until after hours when both you and Rachel can attend to them.

D Suggest that FY1 doctors should be prohibited from going to theatre.

E Talk to Rachel and suggest dividing theatre and ward time more evenly.

13. You overhear a medical student on the bus who is giving a rather unfavourable description of your consultant's clinical competence. You do not believe that it is his intention to be deliberately heard, but it is clear that other passengers are listening.

Rank in order the following actions in response to this situation (1 = Most appropriate; 5 = Least appropriate)

A Explain that the student might have misunderstood the reasons for the consultant's decision.

B Do nothing as it is a public place and medical students are not Trust employees.

C Try to catch the medical student another day to explain that his comments were unhelpful.

D Write a letter to the dean of his medical school.

E Suggest to the student that he exercises caution when talking about colleagues in public.

14. Your registrar frequently undermines your organizational skills on the morning ward round. He expects you to take what you believe is unfair initiative in terms of organizing investigations before the patients are reviewed by a senior member of the team. He also criticizes your note writing and you cannot seem to avoid this, whatever changes you make to your documentation style.

Rank in order the following actions in response to this situation (1 = Most appropriate; 5 = Least appropriate)

A Explain to the registrar privately that you feel that he expects too much initiative from an FY1 doctor.

B Ask the registrar to show you how he would like notes taken on the ward round.

C Inform your consultant that the registrar is constantly belittling your abilities as a doctor.

D Arrange a meeting with Medical Staffing and ask that you are timetabled so as to avoid the registrar as much as possible.

E Ignore your registrar's interpersonal style, but try to accommodate his whims.

15. Each time you phone radiology, you receive a barrage of criticism from a particularly discourteous radiology registrar. Your colleagues now try to make fewer requests whenever this particular registrar is on duty. He once criticized your 'incoherent' radiology requests and when you asked how your requests could be improved, he hung up the phone.

Rank in order the following actions in response to this situation (1 = Most appropriate; 5 = Least appropriate)

A Arrange a meeting between the radiology registrar and the mess president.

B Raise the issue with your Clinical Supervisor.

C Ask for a slot at the monthly radiology meeting to discuss communication between junior doctors and duty registrars.

D Contact the Clinical Director for radiology to explain your difficulty.

E Avoid making radiology requests when this registrar is on duty, unless they are absolutely necessary.

16. Your SHO discloses to you that she is going through a very difficult separation and occasionally has suicidal thoughts.

Choose the THREE most appropriate actions to take in this situation

A Reassure her and tell her that everything will be OK.

B Do not get involved with her personal affairs.

C Offer a friendly ear if and when she wishes to talk further.

D Suggest that she attends counselling.

E Suggest that she books an appointment with her GP.

F Suggest that she speaks to her Educational Supervisor.

G Ask the registrar to prescribe antidepressants.

H Detain her under Section 5(2) of the Mental Health Act 1983.

17. You are reviewing your patients on the ward round, and Mrs Egbert asks if you will need to perform another examination 'down below' as it was uncomfortable yesterday. You cannot understand why this was performed during the SHO's ward round, and the examination had not been detailed in the medical notes.

Choose the THREE most appropriate actions to take in this situation

A Inform the vulnerable adults nurse.

B Inform your consultant.

C Attempt to establish more detail about Mrs Egbert's complaints and the nature of the examination.

D Ask your SHO to describe his review of Mrs Egbert yesterday.

E Speak to the SHO in front of the registrar at the evening handover.

F Contact your Medical Director.

G Inform the patient's family about what has happened.

H Ask the patient not to reveal any information about the incident to anyone else until her consultant has spoken to her.

18. Despite your best efforts, your Educational Supervisor refuses to see you because he is too busy. Eight weeks into your rotation, he eventually asks you to attend theatre and tries to complete your induction meeting between surgical cases but only manages to spend a few minutes talking to you. He concludes your brief encounter by asking you to sign an online educational agreement.

Choose the THREE most appropriate actions to take in this situation

A Sign the agreement, and go home and read it in more detail.

B Do not sign the educational agreement.

C Establish whether it will be possible to arrange a more effective meeting in the near future.

D Ask your favourite consultant to act as your Educational Supervisor instead.

E Ask your clinical supervisor to act as your Educational Supervisor instead.

F Report your Educational Supervisor to the deanery.

G Arrange a meeting with the Foundation Programme Director.

H Persist with future brief meetings.

19. Your registrar asks you to prepare a presentation for the hospital grand round. You are very keen to present at the grand round, although eventually you realize that she intends to present the case in its entirety and merely wants you to do the preparation work.

Rank in order the following actions in response to this situation (1 = Most appropriate; 5 = Least appropriate)

A Ask the registrar if you can present at least part of the case, as it will be good experience.

B Ask the registrar to make a case presentation for you to present the following week.

C Inform your consultant about your registrar's lack of fairness.

D Refuse to hand over the slides for the presentation.

E Do nothing as she is your senior and there has been educational value in producing the slides.

20. Your registrar suffers from reflux disease and is experiencing very bad heartburn after lunch. His symptoms stop him from carrying out the ward round. He informs a nurse he forgot to take his usual proton pump inhibitor (PPI) that morning and is given omeprazole from the drug cabinet.

Rank in order the following actions in response to this situation (1 = Most appropriate; 5 = Least appropriate)

A Report the registrar for taking patient medication.

B Suggest that he obtains the medication from A&E by admitting himself as a patient and having the medicine formally prescribed.

C Offer to prescribe omeprazole for your registrar on a discharge summary prescription.

D Reprimand the nurse who has given him the PPI.

E Do nothing.

21. You overhear a conversation between two of your foundation colleagues Peter and James. Peter describes receiving a police caution the previous weekend during a raucous outing that followed a stressful week of on-call nights. The nature of the offence sounds fairly benign, but it does not seem as if your colleague has any intention of informing anybody else.

Rank in order the following actions in response to this situation (1 = Most appropriate; 5 = Least appropriate)

A Tell Peter that you will be informing the GMC.

B Arrange a meeting with Peter's Educational Supervisor to discuss what you heard.

C Speak to Peter about what you have heard and whether he is aware of the guidance related to receiving cautions.

D Do nothing as the offence sounds relatively benign and no harm has been done.

E Speak to James, and establish more details about the nature of the events.

22. You learn that your colleague is struggling to cannulate patients, despite being in his second FY1 placement.

Rank in order the following actions in response to this situation (1 = Most appropriate; 5 = Least appropriate)

A Help to train your colleague by guiding him through cannulation and practising in the clinical skills laboratory.

B Ignore the problem unless a serious incident occurs.

C Tell your colleague to ask a senior for help.

D Fast-bleep the consultant in order to share your concerns with him.

E Email his Clinical Supervisor.

23. You are assisting a senior registrar in theatre during an inguinal hernia repair. You have seen a lot of hernia repairs during your training, and you are certain that the registrar has inadvertently tied off the vas deferens during this operation. Your registrar denies this, but when you ask him to identify the vas, he does not respond convincingly.

Rank in order the following actions in response to this situation (1 = Most appropriate; 5 = Least appropriate)

A Accept that your registrar is much more experienced and probably correct.

B Ask the anaesthetist to become involved.

C Allow the procedure to be completed before raising the issue with the consultant in charge.

D Insist that the surgeon stops as you are confident that a mistake has been made.

E Leave the operating table and contact the consultant, asking him to attend the theatre.

24. Jill is a specialist nurse on your renal team. She is very knowledgeable, but you feel that she can be overbearing in clinical situations and you frequently feel undermined in your position as a junior doctor.

Choose the THREE most appropriate actions to take in this situation

A Discuss your feelings with Jill and ask how she thinks you could overcome this difficulty.

B Remind Jill of your superior position as a doctor.

C Adopt a more confident approach to patient care.

D Try to gain Jill's respect by finding an opportunity to challenge her clinical judgement and demonstrate your superior knowledge.

E Adopt a more subordinate position as you are less experienced.

F Speak to your senior colleagues for advice.

G Ask the nursing staff whether they find Jill difficult to work with.

H Do nothing as long as her behaviour does not impact on clinical care.

25. Annabelle, the Ward Sister, has bleeped you and asks you to prescribe atenolol to a patient who is hypertensive. After reviewing the patient, you disagree and feel that antihypertensives are not clinically indicated. Annabelle is not convinced by your explanation, saying that, in her 'extensive experience', they are needed.

Rank in order the following actions in response to this situation (1 = Most appropriate; 5 = Least appropriate)

A Explain how and why you arrived at your decision not to prescribe antihypertensives.

B Insist on your management plan as you are responsible for signing the prescription.

C Agree to prescribe antihypertensives, but ask the patient's GP to stop them on discharge.

D Inform Annabelle that you will discuss the issue with a senior colleague but that she should not give any medication for the time being.

E Agree that she should give the medication, but do not sign the prescription chart.

26. Vera is an elderly patient on the orthogeriatrics ward who is currently receiving 20 minutes of counselling a week from the psychologist. After reviewing her, you believe that she might benefit from more regular counselling.

Rank in order the following actions in response to this situation (1 = Most appropriate; 5 = Least appropriate)

A Speak to other multi-disciplinary team members before the weekly meeting to gauge their thoughts.

B Invite Vera and her family to the multi-disciplinary team meeting to voice their concerns.

C Continue with the psychologist's current treatment plan.

D Tell the psychologist he should visit Vera at least twice a week.

E Ask the psychologist whether they think Vera might benefit from additional input.

27. There is a cardiac arrest call in the outpatients clinic at the other side of the hospital. You arrive to find a nurse performing chest compressions, being watched by a domestic assistant and a final-year medical student.

Rank in order the following actions in response to this situation (1 = Most appropriate; 5 = Least appropriate)

A Instruct the medical student to take over chest compressions.

B Encourage the medical student to lead the crash call to develop his leadership skills.

C Instruct the domestic assistant to bring the crash trolley.

D Instruct the medical student to bring the crash trolley, while you take over chest compressions.

E Wait for instructions from the nurse doing compressions.

28. You are planning to review all your patients quickly before the consultant's weekly ward round. The pharmacist insists that you immediately change all your 'as required' prescriptions of paracetamol from '1 g qds' to '500 mg–1 g qds', according to a new Trust guideline. She says that she will have to call your consultant if you do not do this immediately. You have no concerns about your original prescription, and there are 25 patients for whom this would need to be rewritten.

Rank in order the following actions in response to this situation (1 = Most appropriate; 5 = Least appropriate)

A Tell the pharmacist to call your consultant as you have other tasks to complete before the ward round.

B Explain to the pharmacist that there is no substantial difference between the prescriptions but that you will speak to your consultant when he begins the ward round.

C Tell the pharmacist that you will correct your prescription charts immediately.

D Tell the pharmacist that you will return after the ward round, if possible, to complete the task.

E Tell the pharmacist that you will hand this over to the evening team.

29. You are working on a busy surgical on-call shift when you are bleeped for a fifth time by a junior nurse for another 'trivial' task which could wait until the regular team arrives the following day.

Rank in order the following actions in response to this situation (1 = Most appropriate; 5 = Least appropriate)

A Tell her not to phone you again.

B Explain how few doctors are working out of hours and how to decide which jobs require urgent attention.

C Go to the ward and ask the senior nurse to triage all further bleeps.

D Take the referral and add it to your list of tasks.

E Listen to the referral while asking for appropriate details.

30. You are confident that your patient requires an abdominal ultrasound scan, but the radiologist has refused your request twice, initially because of insufficient clinical details and then for unconvincing blood results. Your consultant has insisted that the scan is done today.

Rank in order the following actions in response to this situation (1 = Most appropriate; 5 = Least appropriate)

A Speak to another radiologist.

B Explain that your consultant has examined the patient and, unless the radiologist is willing to do the same, he should accept the request.

C Ask your consultant for advice.

D Take the medical notes and go to speak with the radiologist in person.

E Do not order the ultrasound scan.

31. While working as the surgical FY1 doctor over the weekend, you are asked to complete a discharge letter for a patient whom you have never met. After searching his medical notes, you are unable to find any clear plan for follow-up. The Ward Sister is unsure, and the registrar is in emergency theatre. The patient and his family are insistent on leaving, as they have waited more than four hours for his discharge letter.

Choose the THREE most appropriate actions to take in this situation

A Keep trying to contact your surgical registrar.

B Apologize for the delay and explain that you have been seeing unwell patients for the last few hours.

C Ask the patient to telephone the consultant's secretary in two weeks if he has not received a follow-up appointment.

D Book a routine post-operative clinic appointment with the consultant in six weeks.

E Leave a clear note for the attention of the surgical team, asking them to contact the patient to arrange further follow-up.

F Ask the GP to decide the follow-up.

G Ask the medical registrar for advice.

H Ask the patient to sign a disclaimer stating he is leaving against medical advice.

32. You are trying to arrange two weeks of annual leave in six months' time to attend your friend's wedding abroad. Despite emailing and telephoning the rota coordinator at the hospital where you will be working, you have been unable to secure the time off.

Choose the THREE most appropriate actions to take in this situation

A Write a formal letter of complaint to the hospital.

B Try to arrange cover by swapping your annual leave with a colleague once the rota is published.

C Inform your future Clinical Supervisor that you will be requesting annual leave.

D Send a further email to the rota coordinator, copying in anyone else who might be able to help, such as the human resources representative looking after new foundation doctors.

E Contact a locum agency to assess the cost and availability of cover.

F Do not make any further attempts to arrange your leave for fear of antagonizing the rota coordinator.

G Cancel your plans to attend the wedding.

H Inform your current Clinical Supervisor.

33. After the afternoon surgical ward round, you have amassed a long list of tasks. These include seven venepunctures and an outpatient venesection which was scheduled for an hour ago, two cannulae, and three discharge summaries. You consider how you will complete these tasks.

Rank in order the following actions in response to this situation (1 = Most appropriate; 5 = Least appropriate)

A Bleep the phlebotomy team to ask for assistance while you approach the outpatient venesection.

B Attend the outpatient department where you were scheduled to perform a venesection an hour ago, and then prioritize the other tasks.

C Hand over your list of jobs to the ward nurse and ask her to bleep you if there are any problems.

D Head to the coffee shop with FY1 friends to prioritize your tasks and recruit help if possible.

E Ask another FY1 colleague for help.

34. As the FY1 doctor in gastroenterology, you are arranging the discharge of a patient who is dependent on alcohol and was admitted with symptoms of withdrawal. He has many social problems, including unemployment and long-term disability. In an effort to maintain abstinence from alcohol, you consider the different healthcare professionals you will need to involve, as well as outpatient follow-up with your consultant.

Choose the THREE most appropriate in this situation

A Ward Sister working on the admitting ward.

B GP.

C Drug and alcohol liaison officer.

D Housing assistant.

E Social worker.

F Citizen's Advice Bureau.

G Psychologist.

H Liver transplant services.

35. You are coming to the end of your first FY1 rotation in endocrinology. The job was challenging and you felt inadequately prepared for many of the responsibilities during induction. You consider how you might go about helping your successor.

Rank in order the following actions in response to this situation (1 = Most appropriate; 5 = Least appropriate)

A Feed back your thoughts on the induction to your Clinical Supervisor during your final meeting.

B Write a list of useful tips for your successor.

C Take a week off your next rotation to help support your successor during their first week.

D Leave your mobile phone number for your successor to contact you if they encounter difficulties.

E Leave the induction process to the Foundation Programme management team.

36. Your SHO has a habit of sending text messages on his phone during the ward round. Your consultant has not noticed, but you have seen a number of patients and relatives appear less than impressed with his inattention.

Rank in order the following actions in response to this situation (1 = Most appropriate; 5 = Least appropriate)

A Let the SHO know that others have noticed him sending text messages.

B Ask the SHO whether everything is OK.

C Suggest that the SHO put his phone away immediately.

D Inform the consultant.

E Initiate a 'politeness code', including a rule against excessive texting, which all members of the team should sign.

37. You are working on a busy medical ward which is famously understaffed. Since your new SHO started the rotation two weeks ago, she has left work 45 minutes early every day to collect her children from school. You are working until 8 p.m. most days and still feel that you are not on top of the workload.

Rank in order the following actions in response to this situation (1 = Most appropriate; 5 = Least appropriate)

A Ask her to cover you for the first 45 minutes of your shift.

B Ask her to work during her lunch break to make up the missing time.

C Arrange a meeting with your consultant to discuss her early departure.

D Tell the SHO that you will be informing the consultant unless she is able to make alternative arrangements for the collection of her children.

E Establish whether the childcare arrangements are temporary.

38. Your registrar is known for his strong opinions. As an aside from the ward round, he tells the group of juniors that migrants from Eastern Europe are stretching the NHS to breaking point. You are aware of a Polish patient nearby who is listening intently and appears to be taking offence.

Choose the THREE most appropriate actions to take in this situation

A Apologize to the patient for your registrar's comments.

B Try to move the ward round on to the next patient.

C Challenge the registrar's viewpoint by outlining the contribution immigrants have made to the NHS.

D Agree with the registrar to appease him and move the ward round on.

E Speak to the registrar privately after the ward round about how you felt that the patient was reacting.

F Leave the round to speak to the consultant.

G Share your concerns with the consultant if your registrar does not become more sensitive.

H Return to the patient after the ward round to suggest that they make a formal complaint.

39. A fellow FY1 doctor regularly takes home surgical supplies (e.g. disposable tools and sutures) to practise surgical skills.

Rank in order the following actions in response to this situation (1 = Most appropriate; 5 = Least appropriate)

A Speak to the theatre manager about equipment being taken inappropriately.

B Insist that if your colleague continues to take hospital property you will have to report him.

C Email his Clinical Supervisor with the details.

D Do nothing as it is good that your colleague is practising to become a better doctor.

E Insist that he returns the hospital property immediately.

40. It is the third consecutive week that your SHO has not covered your duties in the preoperative assessment clinic for an hour while you attend mandatory teaching. Each time she has arrived 30 minutes late, despite being given plenty of warning. She always says she has been busy with the ward patients.

Choose the THREE most appropriate actions to take in this situation

A Leave the preoperative assessment clinic with instructions that the SHO should be bleeped if she does not arrive.

B Bleep the registrar and ask her to contact the SHO before each teaching session.

C Inform your Clinical Supervisor that you are not meeting teaching commitments because there is inadequate cover for your absence.

D Ask a colleague to sign you into the teaching and pick up an extra handout.

E Speak to your SHO to identify what is stopping her from arriving and whether her tasks can be reprioritized.

F Email the teaching coordinator to explain your absence.

G Arrange for the nurse specialist to cover your duties for the hour during teaching.

H Ask the clinical secretaries to shorten the preoperative assessment clinics by an hour.

41. An FY1 doctor from a neighbouring ward asks you to hold his bleep because of a personal emergency at home.

Rank in order the following actions in response to this situation (1 = Most appropriate; 5 = Least appropriate)

A Try to prioritize tasks from both wards, and assess whether these can be met before escalation.

B Refuse to hold his bleep until additional support can be guaranteed.

C Inform your registrar.

D Agree to help, provided he does the same for you in the near future.

E Attend your colleague's ward and prioritize his patient's tasks for the rest of the day.

42. You overhear a registrar admonish a student nurse for failing to properly document patient observations. The student nurse later tells you the registrar has shouted at her three times this week for the same issue.

Rank in order the following actions in response to this situation (1 = Most appropriate; 5 = Least appropriate)

A Try to teach the student nurse a better method for recording patient observations.

B Suggest the student nurse explain the situation to her supervisor.

C Speak with your consultant, to establish whether the registrar has any personal problems which explain their behaviour.

D Ask the student nurse to confront the registrar directly if this happens again.

E Formally notify the Matron.

43. You are an FY1 doctor attending a cardiac arrest. You have now attended several emergencies on the same ward and have found one particular nurse standing back, seemingly unsure how to contribute.

Rank in order the following actions in response to this situation (1 = Most appropriate; 5 = Least appropriate)

A Focus on your own performance.

B Stop the crash call and assign everyone specific roles, including the uncertain nurse.

C Suggest to the nurse to begin chest compressions at the next available opportunity during this crash call.

D Tell the nurse to wait outside the bay if they are not participating.

E Ask the nurse to run blood samples to the labs and order X-rays.

44. You diagnose a patient in A&E with a peptic ulcer. You realize your orthopaedic FY1 colleague who discharged the patient 3 months ago mistakenly prescribed her long-term non-steroidal anti-inflammatory drugs (NSAIDs) despite her previous history of gastritis.

Choose the THREE most appropriate actions to take in this situation

A Ignore; it is impossible to attribute one single risk factor as causing a disease.

B Suggest considering litigation against the pharmaceutical company.

C Inform the FY1 doctor responsible.

D Fill out an incident form.

E Discuss with your own consultant.

F Apologize to the patient for the mistake made by your colleague.

G Arrange a teaching session for medical students on the risks of NSAIDs.

H Correct your FY1 colleague's previous discharge letter.

45. You overhear an FY1 colleague explaining his approach for dealing with ward jobs overnight. He asks the nurses to collate all jobs to be completed by 10 p.m. every evening, before turning off his bleep. He explains he can be contacted via his mobile for any peri-arrest, but anything else must wait until the following morning.

Choose the THREE most appropriate actions to take in this situation

A Explain that other tasks less critical than peri-arrest emergencies should still be completed.

B Accept that each FY1 doctor will develop their individualized working practices and that these should be respected, provided emergencies are appropriately dealt with.

C Suggest he extends this deadline to midnight.

D Suggest he should leave his bleep on and allow nurses to judge whether he should be disturbed.

E Speak with the nurses on the ward directly, to assess whether this is causing difficulties for them.

F Inform your colleague's consultant.

G Ask switchboard to forward all bleep requests for your colleague to his mobile phone.

H Attend the hospital on your colleague's night shift to monitor his behaviour.

ANSWERS

1. B, E, D, A, C

All healthcare professionals are in positions of trust and must act within the highest standards of integrity. The porter has made a very serious allegation which could have damaging legal and professional consequences. For this reason, the initial claim justifies some preliminary investigation to broadly establish the facts (B) before informing the Ward Sister. The Ward Sister is a more practical and appropriate port of call than your consultant (E), particularly as she is responsible for the nurses and HCAs on the ward. However, your consultant might have useful advice and would be more appropriate to contact than delegating responsibility for investigating further to the porter (D). (A) and (C) are very incorrect, but (C) is marginally worse as it could represent an even greater over-reaction. Although it may be necessary to call the police later on, this is likely to be handled by hospital security that will have more experience of dealing with similar issues.

2. E, A, D, C, B

It is essential to ensure the safety of patients. However, you should first explain your concerns privately (E) in case a good explanation is forthcoming before asking directly whether your consultant may be under the influence of alcohol (A). If this is admitted or you are not convinced by his denial, you should ensure that he leaves the clinical area. This should be done discreetly, but involving other staff and/or security if necessary. Once the situation has been made safe, you have a duty to escalate the incident to an appropriate person, in this case the Clinical Director (D). Involving other members of staff would only be justifiable if you are insufficiently certain to approach your consultant directly (C) (B). However, these answers are not ideal until the other approaches have been tried unsuccessfully. Escalating to your registrar (who is an immediate senior and probably better known to you) (C) seems more appropriate than contacting your consultant's secretary (B). Even if your concern is justifiable and genuinely held, you should involve as few colleagues as possible to minimize professional embarrassment.

3. A, C, E, D, B

Effective working relationships require individuals to have some discretion about planning their workload. However, the nurse may not appreciate the urgency of the task, which should be reiterated in the first instance. For this reason, the best answer is (A). If a further delay is anticipated, it may be necessary to escalate the issue, as the nurse in charge (C) might intervene or allocate a nurse from elsewhere to help. (E) is correct but not as much as (A) and (C), as you are likely to have other tasks and will not be as familiar with preparing infusions as the nursing staff. It is, however, preferable (if you can do so safely) than *insisting* it is done immediately (D) which may be unsuccessful and risks jeopardizing future working relationships. The worst answer is (B), as you must advocate for your patient and it is not sufficient to satisfy yourself that a drug was prescribed if you know that it has not been administered.

4. C, E, B, D, A

Ideally, discharge summaries should be completed by an individual involved in the patient's care. However, if the outgoing team neglected to complete one, it is important that it is completed to the best of your ability. As you are unfamiliar with the patient and local policy for follow-up, the best answer is to check with a senior colleague who might remember the case (C). This is preferable to blindly arranging a routine appointment in six weeks (E). This would, however, ensure that the patient was not lost to follow-up and might be preferable to asking your SHO to complete the task (B), as they have also rotated posts and are unlikely to add anything further to the discharge summary. Although courtesy requires completing routine tasks before rotating to a new job, it would be inappropriate to expect your predecessor to complete the discharge summary when they are now in a new post and/or hospital. For this reason, (D) and (A) are both incorrect. However, (A) is slightly worse as it puts the ward clerk in the difficult position of having to inappropriately pursue your predecessor after they have moved posts.

5. D, C, A, B, E

Doctors have a duty to act professionally at all times and it would seem that your registrar might have erred in this respect. The best answer is (D), as you should first find out what was overheard to best inform your conversation with the registrar. (C) is also correct, as you should assure the patient that you will raise her concerns, even if she does not wish to make a formal complaint. It is only a 'worse' answer than (D), as you could only really do so with a little more information. Only after completing (D) and (C) should you speak privately to the registrar so that he is aware of the concerns (A). (E) and (B) are incorrect answers. Although (B) would be inappropriate, it is not as destructive as (E) which would be unfair and might either precipitate a formal complaint or reduce the likelihood of her raising concerns in future.

6. D, E, G

If you have concerns with the standard of care given to patients, you have a duty to report them, particularly if patients are potentially at risk. You should not be dissuaded from raising concerns because a doctor is popular (B) or you do not have proof (A). Ideally, concerns of this nature should be raised with the doctor involved in the first instance (D). He might explain his decisions and/or modify his practice without further action being necessary. If advice is needed as to how to proceed, other senior colleagues (E) and/or your Educational Supervisor (G) are appropriate contacts.

Informing the Primary Care Trust (F) or the British Medical Association (H) would be inappropriate, and although a GMC referral might be necessary at some point (C), a concern of this nature might be more effectively dealt with informally.

7. E, C, D, A, B

Clinical incident reporting is important for identifying local error patterns. For this reason, a report should be completed for the 'near miss', even though the patient came to no harm. A clinical incident report (E) is the most appropriate method of error reporting, as it will be dealt with through a formal process and creates a paper trail. (C) is unnecessary, although the lead pharmacist would at least know the correct procedure and ensure you completed a formal incident report. Your consultant *could* be told (D) but is likely to be sent a copy of the incident report, and you do not wish to cause your registrar unnecessary professional embarrassment by raising the issue too often. For this reason, it is worse than (C). Your consultant would, however, correctly direct you to complete an incident form. (A) is the next worst answer, as it implies no attempt to report 'near misses' and hints at covering up a clinical error to protect a colleague. It is, however, perhaps less important, given that the error was corrected at such an early stage. Informing the nursing staff (B) is probably the least helpful response, as it implies no attempt to report the issue formally and potentially undermines your registrar. The only exception might be if this was necessary to stop the dose being administered once it has been crossed off the drug chart.

8. B, A, D, E, C

Multi-disciplinary team meetings are important forums for identifying and solving medical and social problems in conjunction with allied health professional colleagues. It is not necessarily the doctor's responsibility to lead such meetings, but you do have a shared responsibility to ensure that the team is working effectively. In this case, time is being wasted and you should help to facilitate the team arrive at a decision. The best response is (B), as the nurse should be given space to voice her concerns uninterrupted and it might yet be possible to resolve the disagreement. An alternative approach would be to revisit the case later on (A), so that it can be addressed with fresh minds and progress can be made through the agenda. However, this might simply postpone the disagreement and risks the case being forgotten or not considered for lack of time. For this reason, it is not as good an answer as (B).

Although the social worker might have an opinion, she has not contributed so far and this might suggest that she has nothing specific to add (D). For this reason, it is not as good a strategy as (B) and (A), although an additional perspective could help. It is probably incorrect to leave the nurse and occupational therapist to resolve their differences (E), as they have not made any progress alone so far. The worst answer is (C), as it is not your place to ask anyone to leave the meeting, and this would be the wrong time to lose the occupational therapist's expertise.

9. D, C, A, B, E

Personality clashes and differences in approach are inevitable consequences of multi-disciplinary teamworking. However, these must not be allowed to impact on patient care. Although neither surgeons nor physiotherapists are necessarily 'correct' about optimal mobilization arrangements, consensus is more likely to follow collaborative working. The best answer is (D), as a senior colleague might have a better understanding of the situation and might be able to suggest a way forward. (C) might be a positive development but might be better suggested by someone other than the FY1 doctor—your senior colleague might help. For this reason, (D) is preferable to (C). It is always helpful to involve other members of the multi-disciplinary team (e.g. nurses and occupational therapists) in discharge arrangements, so that a consensus is established before meetings take place (A). However, this is worse than (D) and (C), as it risks alienating the physiotherapist and making her feel as if the outcome of meetings has been determined without her beforehand.

(B) and (E) are the two wrong answers. Asking for the physiotherapist to be replaced (B) is likely to damage working relationships, and this is rarely the place of a junior doctor rotating temporarily through a post. However, (E) is the worst answer, as you cannot blindly accept the physiotherapist's advice when this conflicts with that of your consultant. Mobilization arrangements will depend on operative considerations (e.g. bone quality, fracture pattern, and choice of metalwork), details to which the physiotherapist may not have access. The consultant is ultimately responsible for patient care and should be informed if his instructions are routinely being disregarded.

10. B, E, A, C, D

Handover between teams must be done correctly to ensure that important tasks are not missed. This is particularly vital, given current employment regulations which have made shift working more commonplace.

As this issue relates to a group of doctors, the best answer is (B) which would allow you to assess the degree of support that you have for change and collect helpful suggestions. Informing a senior consultant might lead to change more quickly but could alternatively lead to no change at all, depending on the individual concerned. As a handover meeting is already scheduled but being used inadequately, it would be preferable to address the problem with your colleagues, if possible, (B) before approaching a senior colleague (E) to suggest changes, for example starting the handover meeting at an earlier time. Your own handover should already be effective (A), but this might be hindered if there are adverse structural issues such as other doctors wanting you to hurry up. In this case, the culture of accepting poor-quality handovers must be challenged. For this reason, (A) is a worse answer than (B) and (E), as it does not address the wider problem. (C) and (D) are wrong answers. Submitting incident reports for many different doctors (C) will make you unpopular. Although it might result in change, it risks creating a personal issue out of a cultural problem and would not be a measured response to your problem. There is no such thing as a 'routine' task—either it needs to be done or it does not. Even checking a 'routine' blood test is important if the patient is found to be severely hyperkalaemic. Doing nothing (D) in this case is the worst option.

11. D, B, E, A, C

You should be aware of factors that might cause colleagues to under-perform, including poor health. As Frances has confided in you, it would seem appropriate to ask how she feels (D) and whether she is cop-ing. This is a fairly uncontroversial answer and is undoubtedly the best in this case. Ideally, she should let her Educational Supervisor know in case anything can be done, or must be done in future, to support her at work (B). (B) is not as good as (D), simply because you are likely to solicit more information discreetly before proffering advice. (E) is cor-rect, although not as good as (D) and (B) in isolation, as your immediate concern should be to acknowledge the information Frances has chosen to share. The two worst answers are (A) and (C). Although Frances may benefit from counselling (A), you cannot presume that this is something she would want. The worst answer is of course (C), as it would not be your place to tell other people about Frances' health unless there is evi-dence of her underperforming and putting patients at risk.

12. E, B, D, A, C

As foundation doctors, both you and Rachel are expected to gain spe-cific competencies. Rachel is at risk of not doing this effectively. Similarly, as an FY1 doctor on a surgical placement, you should assist in theatre if there is time available, as this is also relevant experience. Although it is reasonable to divide tasks according to your respective interests, you should both aim to gain experience of each setting.

The best answer is usually to try to resolve problems locally first, in this case by speaking to Rachel (E). Trying to alter her behaviour by achieving consensus is preferable to *insisting* she spends more time on the ward (B), which might be unsuccessful and risks souring your rela-tionship. (D) is also unnecessarily confrontational and additionally risks limiting both FY1 doctors' exposure to an important part of their surgi-cal experience. As usual, doing nothing when presented with a problem (A) ranks poorly and you should not accept such a stark discrepancy without challenge. (C) is, however, clearly the worst answer, as leaving tasks until after hours means both FY1 doctors routinely staying late and risks either inconveniencing patients or exposing them to danger.

13. E, A, C, D, B

Your first step should be to stop the medical student continuing this con-versation in public, as colleagues (like patients) are entitled to a degree of privacy. The best way to achieve this would be to let the student know he can be overheard and that this is unacceptable (E). It is likely that most students would respond to such a warning, even away from a teaching environment. Although (A) achieves a similar goal of letting the student know he has been overheard, it is a worse option as it risks entering a debate about your consultant's ability. (C) is not as good as (E) and (A), as it does not stop the conversation, although it might address the student's long-term behaviour. (D) is incorrect, as it is an overescala-tion of a situation that could be more appropriately resolved in other ways. You might contact the medical school dean if you became aware of more serious concerns regarding a student, e.g. cheating or criminal activity. However, (D) is not as bad as (B) because the medical school dean would probably forward your concern to a more appropriate person (e.g. the student's personal tutor), which would lead to the issue being addressed. (B) is the worst answer, as it does not help the medical student (who needs guidance), your consultant (who needs support in his absence), and other passengers (whose trust in the medical profession might be damaged).

14. A, B, E, C, D

Mutual respect is essential to any effective professional relationship. Your registrar might not realize how unconstructive his style has become and he might improve if approached directly. For this reason, (A) is the best answer. Asking his advice about note taking might help reduce confrontation (B), and this answer is only less correct as it seems you have already made considerable effort to adapt your style. (E) is similar to (B) but is a worse answer, as it does not demonstrate to your registrar that you are trying hard to understand how to improve. (C) and (D) are incorrect, at least initially, as they represent premature escalation of your difficulties which are best resolved in other ways. (D) is only worse, as it is a more significant escalation than (C).

15. B, D, C, A, E

The NHS employs 1.4 million people, some of whom have challenging personalities. However, if junior doctors are dissuaded from requesting investigations because of an obstructive radiologist, this has to be addressed. As you are unlikely to know the registrar and work in a different department, you should initially escalate the issue up your own hierarchy first (B). (D) is a worse answer, as it represents a bold step and would be best done with the support of your Clinical or Educational Supervisor. The remaining answers are incorrect. Although (C) addresses the issue, opening a dialogue in such a public forum is inappropriate when your concerns are about a specific colleague. It is, however, a better option than (A), as the mess president is unlikely to contribute very much. The worst answer has to be (E), as your clinical judgement should not be swayed by an impolite colleague who would risk patient safety.

16. C, E, F

It is important for medical professionals to ensure their own personal health and well-being. In this scenario, your SHO has revealed a serious psychological symptom which needs to be addressed (B). This might be alleviated through some form of counselling (D) or with antidepressants (G), although she initially requires a full medical assessment by an independent and objective healthcare professional (E). Professionally, she may benefit from the advice and support of her Educational Supervisor who has responsibility for her pastoral care (F). It is also reasonable to offer your own time and attention if she feels that she can speak freely to you (C), but you should avoid false reassurances (A). (H) is incorrect because Section 5(2) of the Mental Health Act 1983 is only applicable to hospital inpatients; your colleague is not at immediate risk, and this action seems unlikely to help nurture a professional working relationship.

17. **B, C, D**

All health professionals have a duty to protect their patients, and we should always be aware of the potential risk to children and vulnerable adults. Nevertheless, we also have a duty to respect our colleagues, and in this scenario, it would be inappropriate to raise a serious concern in front of an unnecessary audience (E) without first establishing more information (C) and speaking to the SHO privately, as there may be a legitimate explanation (D). It is likely that your concerns will need escalation to your consultant (B), who might involve more senior colleagues if necessary, although this would not usually be something an FY1 doctor would organize themselves (A) (F). Informing the patient's family before establishing all the facts is premature and risks unnecessarily compromising the patient's trust if unfounded (G). If a serious assault has occurred, this would be managed by much more senior doctors and the hospital management. However, no doctor should conspire to silence patients and therefore should avoid telling patients what they can and cannot say (H).

18. **B, C, G**

Your Educational Supervisor has responsibility for providing appropriate supervision. This includes finding time for regular meetings. The scenario suggests that you have made substantial efforts to make alternative arrangements, without any meaningful success (H). You might wish to try again to arrange a more effective meeting (C); otherwise it appears reasonable to initiate the process of finding a suitable replacement (G). It would be irresponsible to sign an educational (or any other) agreement without being aware of its contents (A) (B). It is not your responsibility to ask another consultant to take over the role of Educational Supervisor (D) (E), and involving the deanery would not be a measured response at this stage (F).

19. **A, E, B, D, C**

As a junior trainee, your control over a project may not always correlate with your efforts. This should not preclude you from striving for fairness. In this instance, your hard work might be compensated with the chance to present some of your work, and so (A) is the best answer. Although there is value in preparing a presentation, doing nothing is only an option if you are somehow acknowledged in the presentation, to avoid the charge of dishonesty (E). This would still be a more measured response than those remaining.

(B) is incorrect as it is probably unreasonable to expect your registrar to prepare a presentation for you the following week, although this might lead to genuine collaboration on further presentations. However, it would not be as bad as refusing to share your slides (D) or, worse, escalating unnecessarily to your consultant (C).

20. B, C, D, A, E

Doctors should not treat themselves, and taking medication from a drug cupboard is likely to contravene Trust policy. Ideally, the registrar should book in to A&E for an objective assessment, if necessary, to obtain a prescription drug (B). Although this is the best option, it might not be practical and you could alternatively prescribe omeprazole if you are willing to accept responsibility for the prescription (C). However, you should recall that symptoms of heartburn might indicate more serious pathology. (D) is a less positive step than suggesting the earlier alternative approaches, particularly as it is your registrar, and not the nurse, who has instigated this dilemma. However, speaking to those involved is preferable to escalating them prematurely (A). Doing nothing is, as usual, an unacceptable response (E).

21. C, B, A, E, D

GMC guidance states that all doctors must declare any caution or criminal conviction received anywhere in the world. Your professional relationship is most likely to be preserved by speaking to Peter and encouraging him to inform the GMC himself (C), or (less good) via his Educational Supervisor (B), before you consider declaring it yourself (A). Speaking to James will not change the situation, as any caution that is received must be declared, irrespective of the nature of the criminal offence (E). For this reason, (E) is a worse answer than the three which involve someone informing the GMC. (D) is last, as it contravenes GMC guidance and misses an opportunity to help your colleague ensure he does not find himself in additional trouble later on.

22. A, C, E, B, D

It is not obvious from this scenario that there is any immediate danger to patients, although cannulation is a fundamental skill for any junior doctor, and your colleague must learn to master it quickly. Hence, if it is possible to train him to cannulate effectively yourself, with minimal disruption to your duties, this should be attempted in the first instance (A). Although taking responsibility yourself (A) is preferable, seeking senior guidance might also be appropriate, in which case it is better to encourage your colleague to seek help (C), rather than impose it upon him (E). (B) is incorrect but is unlikely to cause serious harm, as people learn skills at different rates and others are also in a position to help your colleague. The worst answer in this case is (D), as the problem is not one that could be resolved immediately, and it does not warrant fast-bleeping your consultant.

23. D, E, B, C, A

This is a very challenging situation, which depends on a number of factors, particularly how confident you are that a mistake has been made and whether this can be reversed if correctly identified intraoperatively. This is an issue of patient safety and you have a duty to raise concerns immediately to ensure the best possible chance of rectifying the error. The best person with whom to raise your concern initially is the operating surgeon, in this case the registrar (D). (E) addresses the problem intraoperatively but leaves the surgeon unassisted and could be very embarrassing if your concerns prove unfounded. For this reason, it is worse than (D). (B) ranks lower because the anaesthetist is unlikely to have seen what happened or to want to become involved in any disagreement. However, they are a senior doctor and might contribute, e.g. by insisting that the consultant surgeon attends the operating theatre. However, waiting until after the operation (C) is worse if your opinion was strongly held, as the immediate opportunity to rectify the error will have been missed. (A) is, of course, unacceptable as you must speak out if you believe a serious error has occurred.

24. A, C, F

Although Jill probably brings a wealth of knowledge and experience to the team, it is also important to foster a positive environment in which all members of the team are respected. It may not immediately impact on patient care, but, indirectly, poor working relationships are likely to lead to less efficient care in the long term and so the issue should be addressed (A) (H). Effective work within a multi-disciplinary team requires mutual respect, rather than trying to establish dominance or accepting subordination (B) (D) (E). Nevertheless, your position of equal worth within the team may be reiterated by adopting a more confident approach (C). Asking the nursing staff whether they find Jill difficult to work with is a leading question, implies fault, and is unlikely to gain you favour with her colleagues (G). In any challenging scenario, it is rarely incorrect to approach a senior colleague for advice (F).

25. D, A, B, C, E

Your response to Annabelle's request must balance exercise of your clinical judgement with maintaining an effective working relationship. Given Annabelle's confidence in her judgement and the fact that she has not accepted your initial explanation, it may be sensible (and diplomatic) to discuss her concerns with a senior colleague at a convenient time (D). (A) is ranked lower only because it seems some attempt has already been made to explain your decision-making. Nevertheless, (A) is better than (B) as *insisting* seems unlikely to nurture a harmonious working relationship with an important colleague. (C) and (E) are both incorrect answers, as you should never prescribe a drug that you do not believe is indicated. Prescribing them initially but stopping them later on (C) would be deceptive and confusing for the patient. However, the worst answer is (E), as you should never suggest that a drug is administered without a prescription.

26. E, A, C, B, D

You should respect the ability of colleagues to deliver their own special-ist services and manage their workload. However, this must be balanced with a duty to advocate for your patient.

In this case, you should speak to the psychologist to determine whether they are happy with their current input (E). They might agree or give reasons as to why so little time is being spent with Vera (e.g. volume of patients requiring attention or staffing pressures). (A) is also an accept-able approach, although (E) is better as the psychologist would be more likely to have an informed opinion than other members of the team. You could certainly accept the psychologist's plan (they are likely to know best), but you have a duty to speak up if you think care could be improved, and so (C) is worse than (E) and (A).

(B) and (D) are incorrect. Although patients can sometimes attend multi-disciplinary team meetings (B), this is unusual and probably inappropriate as other patients are usually discussed as well. In addition, we are given no indication that Vera wants to attend or has indicated any concern about the amount of psychologist input she is receiving. However, the last answer is (D), as it is not your place to instruct the psychologist and such an intervention would probably not be well received.

27. D, A, C, E, B

The most appropriate person arriving at a cardiac arrest should assume the role of team leader. In most cases, this will be the most senior doc-tor present, even if that person is an FY1 doctor. A cardiac arrest should be managed according to established protocols. However, whether the arrest is successful depends, in part, on how well it is led and whether each team member's skills are optimally utilized.

In this case, the best answer is (D), as the nurse is likely to be exhausted at this point (possibly delivering ineffective compressions) and the stu-dent should know what a crash trolley looks like. (A) is an acceptable alternative, although there may be insufficient time to confirm that the student is confident giving compressions and has good technique. (C) unfairly assumes that the domestic assistant would recognize a crash trolley and does not ensure relief of the nurse delivering chest com-pressions. As effective chest compressions are one of the most impor-tant components of managing a cardiac arrest, (C) is ranked lower than (D) and (A). (E) is incorrect, as you should usually (unless the nurse is exceptionally qualified, e.g. critical care outreach or a resuscitation officer) take responsibility for the situation. However, the worst answer is (B), as it would be inappropriate to encourage a student (particularly one you do not know) to lead the resuscitation effort.

28. B, D, A, C, E

The pharmacist's request appears unnecessary and at best non-urgent. Other healthcare professionals should not generally attempt to priori-tize your work, as no one else can fully appreciate the pressures on you at any one time. However, as the pharmacist is concerned, you should offer to raise the issue with a senior colleague at the first convenient opportunity (B). An alternative approach would be to offer to complete the task later on (D), and this is only ranked lower because the task is non-urgent and you cannot guarantee that your priorities will not have changed by the end of the ward round. The pharmacist is unlikely to call your consultant to demand completion of a non-urgent task. However, challenging her to do so (A) would be incorrect, as it risks escalating the situation and embroiling your consultant unnecessarily in the dispute. Nevertheless, this might be preferable to (C), which could mean neglecting important tasks (e.g. reviewing your patients so that the consultant can make better plans on his ward round) to keep the pharmacist happy. The worst answer is (E), as the on-call team is unlikely to be available for routine tasks, which risk distracting them from more urgent demands on the team's time.

29. **E, B, D, C, A**

You must balance your workload against the risk of dissuading the nurse from bleeping doctors in future. The best answer is (E), as you are obliged to listen to the nurse so that she can be satisfied that you have all the details and to ensure that this really is another inappropriate bleep. It may, however, become appropriate to modify her expectations at some point (B), as she is possibly unaware of the skeleton medical team available out of hours, and this might be a valuable education point. (B) is worse than (E), as it is more important to listen and understand the nurse's concern than to emphasize her inappropriate bleeping. Agreeing to complete an inappropriate task (D) risks neglecting other responsibilities and does not address the misunderstanding of which tasks need escalating to a doctor out of hours. For this reason, it is a less helpful response than (E) and (B). Senior nurses sometimes triage bleeps to reduce pressure on the medical team out of hours. However, if this is not already local policy, you risk antagonizing the ward staff by suggesting it (C) at this point. The worst answer is (A), as next time it might be a genuine emergency.

30. **C, D, A, B, E**

The radiologist must also be satisfied that an investigation is indicated before agreeing that it should take place. This can lead to difficulties, as the most junior person on the team (who probably has the least understanding of why the scan is necessary) is often expected to communicate with the radiology consultant.

The best answer is (C), as your consultant might clarify his particular reason for needing an ultrasound scan or think of a different approach to the same problem. (D) is a less appropriate response and will only help if you are armed with additional information—simply harassing the radiologist to accept your request is unlikely to succeed. However, (A) is incorrect as it is bad form to speak to another consultant as a way of skirting a decision made by their colleague. (A) is only marginally better than (B) if only because the latter is unlikely to succeed and may jeopardize any future working with this radiologist. The worst answer is (E), as simply accepting the radiologist's refusal without informing your team risks your patient's well-being by depriving them of a potentially important investigation.

31. **B, C, E**

Although a discharge summary is clinically non-urgent, the patient has already been put to some inconvenience waiting for it to be completed. The regular team should have anticipated a weekend discharge and already completed the paperwork.

You should certainly apologize for the delay so that it is clear that the wait was necessary (B). You could complete the discharge summary from the notes to the best of your ability, but ask the regular team to make arrangements for follow-up (E). This will prevent the patient from having to attend an appointment unnecessarily or being prematurely discharged from surgical care. Although asking the patient to contact the team (C) might challenge his faith in the system, it is an honest approach and adds another layer of reassurance that follow-up will take place.

As the discharge summary is clinically non-urgent, you should not interrupt the surgical registrar in theatre (A). Neither the medical registrar (G) nor the GP (F) should be expected to determine the appropriateness of surgical follow-up. A routine follow-up appointment (D) might ensure further contact with the surgical team but may unnecessarily waste everyone's time.

The patient should not be asked to self-discharge (H), as the only reason for him to remain in hospital is administrative.

32. **B, C, D**

Booking annual leave in advance can be difficult, as rotas are not published and you might not be currently based at the hospital concerned. However, this should not be an impenetrable barrier and you are entitled to make annual leave requests in advance (F) (G). You should aim to let all appropriate people at the hospital know your intention so that workforce arrangements can be made. These people are likely to include (at a minimum) your new Clinical Supervisor (C) and the rota coordinator (D). Once the rota is published, you will be responsible for arranging to swap any on-call shifts (B).

Your current Clinical Supervisor is unlikely to have very much influence, particularly if your leave request involves a different hospital (H). A formal letter of complaint (A) is unlikely to have much impact, might antagonize future colleagues, and will not change the annual leave policy. It is not your responsibility to arrange locum cover for any shifts that you might miss (E).

33. **A, E, B, C, D**

The two most important qualities of an FY1 doctor are effective communication skills and an ability to prioritize. (A) is the best answer, as informing the phlebotomy team about your dilemma early on increases the likelihood of them being able to help. Similarly, another FY1 doctor might be willing to help (E), although this is less ideal as they are likely to have their own tasks to complete. Both answers are, however, better than (B) as they might save you from falling behind on other tasks later if others are able to help.

(C) and (D) are incorrect. It would be inappropriate, and unlikely to foster positive working relationships, if you were to hand over your tasks to the ward team (C). However, you might enlist the help of nurses who are able to take blood if they are available to do so. Although it is worth taking a few minutes to prioritize tasks, taking a coffee break at this point (D) would waste time and risk leaving a patient waiting unnecessarily in the outpatient department. For this reason, (D) is ranked last.

34. B, C, E

Your patient may benefit from all manner of services, but you must balance this against the appropriateness of each referral.

The patient's GP (B) will provide long-term follow-up and will be able to access many different services of potential benefit to your patient. He may also require specialist drug and alcohol input which can be provided by an appropriately qualified person (C). A social worker (E) could also help assess the patient's need for additional services.

The Ward Sister is not likely to expect continued involvement with this man, unless he becomes an inpatient again (A). Similarly, there is no reason to think that he would benefit substantially from housing services (D), the Citizen's Advice Bureau (F), a psychologist (G), or the transplant service (H). These may become necessary in future, which is all the more reason to ensure that he remains engaged with key people such as his GP and social services.

35. A, B, D, E, C

Handover is not only important between shifts, but it is also necessary when moving jobs. You should endeavour to leave all routine tasks completed and a clear set of instructions for your successor.

If there are ways of improving the induction process, you should let an appropriate person (e.g. your Clinical Supervisor) know (A). They will provide continuity between trainees and are best placed to ensure the induction process is improved, based on your feedback. (B) is also appropriate, so your successor inherits your hard-won tips such as schedules and useful bleep numbers. (B) is ranked lower than (A) only because an improved induction process will ensure benefits for trainees at every stage, not just your immediate successor. (D) is a great idea but, in isolation, cannot be better than (B) or (A).

(E) and (C) are both incorrect. (E) is unhelpful, as the Foundation Programme cannot provide the post-specific advice that is likely to be most useful to your successor. It therefore misses an opportunity to help your successor and their patients. (C) is the worst answer because it is excessive, defeats the purpose of annual leave (rest and recuperation!), and perhaps most importantly would disrupt your new team which would have to cope without its FY1 doctor in the first week.

36. **B, A, C, D, E**

Although people will have different priorities, a minimum standard of professional behaviour is expected of all doctors. It is usually possible to enforce this (largely unwritten) code of behaviour informally. In this case, the transgression is relatively minor and so calls for a measured approach. (B) is the best answer, as it raises the issue discreetly in a way that would allow your SHO to modify his behaviour without embarrassment. There may actually be a problem (e.g. an emergency at home) and he might elect to leave the ward round. (A) is ranked lower than (B), as it is more direct and *could* lead to defensiveness in some colleagues. (C) ranks lower than (A) for the same reason, i.e. it is excessively direct. (D) and (E) are incorrect, as they are not measured responses to a relatively minor problem. (E) is particularly excessive and is unlikely to garner much support from other members of your clinical team.

37. **E, D, C, B, A**

In any difficult situation involving colleagues, it is important to establish the facts early on. For this reason, (E) is the best answer. You might be willing to help out your SHO if there is a temporary problem with childcare, but she will be working normal hours in the near future. However, it might become necessary to confront the SHO and make it clear that you are unwilling to accept the current arrangement (D) which risks patient safety and your own well-being. (D) is ranked lower, as (E) is more likely to resolve the issue to everyone's satisfaction without causing unnecessary ill feeling. (C) may become necessary later on but is a worse initial response than (D). If the matter cannot be resolved through discussion, it must be escalated to your consultant. (B) is the first wrong answer. Although time might be made up elsewhere, working through lunch is not an optimal long-term strategy and should not be imposed on the SHO, particularly by the FY1 doctor. The worst answer is (A), as it leaves only one doctor on site for 1.5 hours every day.

38. **B, E, G**

The immediate goal should be to de-escalate what could become an inflammatory situation if an argument were to develop. Your best move would be to steer the ward round back to its original business of reviewing patients (B). However, you should also let the registrar know afterwards that his behaviour raised concerns (E). If this is unsuccessful, the matter should be raised with your consultant (G).

You should avoid becoming embroiled in controversial discussions when these are likely to cause offence in the workplace. This includes agreeing (D) or disagreeing (C) with the registrar.

It would be an over-reaction to leave the ward round (F) or apologize on your registrar's behalf (A), although he might wish to approach the patient after you have brought the issue to his attention. Similarly, you should not usually solicit complaints from patients about colleagues (H).

39. **E, B, A, C, D**

Dishonest removal of hospital equipment constitutes theft, with its attendant legal and professional consequences. The situation would be much different if he had asked an appropriate person (e.g. theatre coordinator) and been given equipment with which to practise. The best answer is (E), as you should give your colleague an opportunity to recognize his actions were incorrect (he might not have thought through the consequences thoroughly) and return any remaining equipment. (B) is correct but would be unnecessarily confrontational as an initial response.

You might wish to let the theatre manager know that property is going missing (A), so that items can be appropriately secured and warnings distributed to staff. However, (A) is not as good as (E) or (B), as it does not directly address the person responsible.

Reporting your colleague outright (C) under these circumstances seems excessive, as it is likely he has not thought through the consequences and does not view his behaviour as stealing. If he had stolen something more obvious (e.g. a hospital computer), you would clearly have to involve the hospital authorities early on.

The worst answer is (D). Although a surgical registrar could perhaps argue that the Trust should make reasonable allowances for practice, this argument is rather less convincing for an FY1 doctor. Instead, he is forcing his employer to subsidize his further professional education without their agreement.

40. **C, E, F**

Attending a set number of teaching sessions is a mandatory requirement for completion of FY1. If you identify difficulties attending sessions, these must be raised early on so that you do not find yourself in difficulty towards the end of the year.

You could certainly speak with the SHO to emphasize the importance of sufficient cover, so that you can attend teaching (E). However, the issue should be escalated swiftly if it persists. Your Clinical Supervisor (C) is a good place to start, followed by your Educational Supervisor if issues are still not resolved. It would also be polite to inform the teaching coordinator as well by way of apology for not arriving (F). You should not leave the clinic without cover, particularly if you doubt that your SHO will arrive on time (A). Similarly, you should not delegate to another healthcare professional (G), unless this has been agreed locally. The secretaries are unlikely to be able to manipulate the clinic volume without impacting on the elective operating list (H). Involving a senior doctor for the simple task of reminding your SHO is unlikely to be received well (B). Asking a colleague to sign you in to teaching casts doubt on both your own and your colleague's probity (D).

41. **A, C, B, D, E**

Your priorities should be to help your colleague at a difficult time while ensuring the patients are adequately cared for. This is best achieved by (A), i.e. clinical prioritization, followed by escalation when appropriate. (C) is also a strong answer, as the registrar will probably suggest following (A) and it is important that others in the hierarchy are aware of unexpected changes to the team. (B) might have been the correct answer, depending on the circumstances, particularly whether or not you can safely manage both wards. The stem does not give any information to suggest that this would be unsafe, particularly if only for a short period of time. If the stem had provided additional hints, e.g. you are 'busy' or the wards were 'large', then (B) might have been the best answer.

Option (D) is sub-optimal, as short-term assistance should not be contingent on reciprocity. (E) is the worst answer, as it suggests neglecting your own patients in order to help your colleague.

42. **B, C, E, A, D**

Unfortunately, you will encounter unprofessional behaviour at some stage during the Foundation Programme. This is perhaps more likely to be observed between members of staff than between staff and patients. In this case, the student nurse might well be uncertain about how to act and cowed by the power dynamic involving a senior member of the medical team. In this case, the best option is to encourage and empower the student nurse to seek advice from her own supervisor (B). Seeking advice from your consultant (C) and informally notifying the Matron (E) might be appropriate if you are concerned that this behaviour is persistent or particularly serious. Your own consultant is likely to be a more appropriate avenue than the Matron, which is why (C) was ranked above (E).

(A) does not really solve the main issue, which is inappropriate behaviour by a professional colleague. (D) is unlikely to be helpful advice, as some people are naturally more assertive than others and this risks aggravating the situation further.

43. **A, E, C, D, B**

In an emergency situation, your focus should be entirely on effective patient care (A). Once the crash call is running optimally, your focus may extend to include secondary training issues. One means of increasing this nurse's confidence might be to actively involve the nurse by delegating tasks (E). (C) is also a task that could be delegated carefully to an uncertain team member. However, (E) is a better answer in this context, as it would be preferable to warn the nurse in advance of asking them to become heavily involved, or at least to confirm that they are confident with basic life support.

(D) is likely to demoralize the nurse unnecessarily, as well as depriving him of the opportunity to learn by observing. It may sometimes be necessary to move staff members away, e.g. if a prolonged arrest is ongoing in a small side room, but this is not mentioned in the question stem

(B) is the worst answer, as stopping the crash call while roles are assigned is dangerous—chest compressions should only be stopped briefly for intermittent ventilations, shocks, and rhythm checks.

44. **C, D, E**

It is important to be able to feed the incident back to your colleague for their benefit (C). It may also need to be reported formally as an incident, so that such events can be monitored and acted upon (D). This will depend on the circumstances. For example, if the risk of gastric ulceration was actively considered, discussed with the patient, and documented; this would be a very different situation to one in which NSAIDs were just prescribed routinely. If there is any doubt, it would be wise to seek senior advice about how best to proceed (E).

The other options are dishonest (H), do not solve the problem at hand (A) (B) (G), or risk undermining your colleague unnecessarily (F).

45. **A, D, E**

The other FY1 doctor's approach clearly is not appropriate, as many 'routine' tasks may need to be completed overnight to ensure that patients are kept safe. This clearly needs to be challenged (A) (D). Speaking with the nurses on the ward will enable you to establish how much the FY1 doctor's approach reflects the reality of his care (E). This might help if it becomes necessary to escalate things later on.

It is not acceptable to overlook this risk to patients (B) (C), to become complicit in the other FY1 doctor's approach (G), or to embark on an extensive investigation of your own (H). It may become necessary to escalate the issue (F), but (A), (D), and (E) are preferable approaches in the first instance.

Section 3

Practice test

Practice test

This chapter presents two practice tests with a mix of question types (e.g. multiple choice or ranking), content (e.g. domain-tested), and styles (e.g. patient, colleague, or personal). Each includes 30 questions and broadly reflects the type of questions likely to be asked in the SJT (p. 7). To make the most of this test, you should complete it in one sitting within an hour before checking your answers (pp. 261–262).

When checking your answers to ranking questions, remember that credit is still given for 'near misses' and so there is no need to hit the 'correct' sequence every time.

The practice test answers are not accompanied by detailed explanations. For this reason, it would be preferable to complete all the questions in Section 2 (pp. 29–230) before attempting the test.

To replicate the SJT as closely as possible, you should ideally complete these questions within an hour under formal examination conditions. Once you have attempted all the questions, turn to p. 261 to check your answers. It is difficult to interpret your final score, as your rank will depend entirely on how well your colleagues (and every other medical student in the country) fare.

If you are organized, you could arrange a study group to work through this book and/or complete the practice test. Marking your answers as a group will give some indication as to your performance relative to others. It will also provide an opportunity to discuss the various options (including disagreement with our answers) and so gain a deeper understanding of the issues tested by the SJT.

QUESTIONS

First exam

1. You are working as an FY1 doctor in the Medical Assessment Unit, seeing Marcin who is a 35-year-old Polish man with very limited English language skills.

Rank in order the following actions in response to this situation (1 = Most appropriate; 5 = Least appropriate)

A Attempt a brief history using hand gestures and diagrams.

B Try to contact a member of Marcin's family to act as an interpreter over the phone.

C Do not attempt a history without a translator present.

D Skip the history, and focus your management on the examination and investigations.

E Extrapolate a history based on the limited findings of the ambulance crew on their initial assessment sheet.

2. During a GP rotation, you see Carl, who would like to know the results of a colonoscopy and CT scan after a joint MDT meeting. He missed his last appointment but has been told that the GP should have access to the report. The results identify a disseminated colorectal malignancy, although no treatment plan has yet been decided upon.

Rank in order the following actions in response to this situation (1 = Most appropriate; 5 = Least appropriate)

A Establish what the patient understands about his diagnosis first.

B Refer him back to the gastroenterologist who performed the colonoscopy.

C Contact the nurse specialist and ask her to telephone the patient as soon as possible.

D Explain the very poor outcome associated with cancers like the one Carl has.

E Ask the patient to come back and see you in the afternoon, as you will need to speak to his hospital doctors first.

3. During a busy urology ward round with your consultant, the nurse mentions that Frank, who is recovering from a transurethral resection of the prostate, has admitted to feeling low over the last few months.

Choose the THREE most appropriate actions to take in this situation

A Ask the consultant to speak to Frank about his low mood.

B Speak to Frank after the ward round.

C Ask Frank if he is low enough for antidepressants.

D Break away from the ward round to discuss the matter with Frank.

E Ask the nurse to keep any additional patient information until the end of the ward round to avoid future interruptions.

F Inform your seniors after the ward round, if a referral needs to be made.

G Tell the patient to speak to someone about his low mood.

H Inform the on-call psychiatrist.

4. You are asked to see Jerry, a 55-year-old man who has recently undergone a colonic resection with defunctioning colostomy. He wishes to make a complaint against the operating consultant, as he feels that he was not adequately informed about the impact of his stoma.

Rank in order the following actions in response to this situation (1 = Most appropriate; 5 = Least appropriate)

A Inform the patient that you will relay his concerns to the consultant.

B Apologize on the consultant's behalf.

C Establish the difficulties that Jerry has been having with the stoma.

D Defend the consultant by explaining that the formation of a stoma was documented on the consent form.

E Inform the patient of the complaints procedure and how he might go about registering a complaint.

5. Your registrar shouts at a medical student in front of a patient. The medical student comes to find you afterwards in tears and is uncertain how to react to this treatment.

Rank in order the following actions in response to this situation (1 = Most appropriate; 5 = Least appropriate)

A Suggest that the student reports the registrar to an appropriate person within the medical school.

B Bleep your registrar and ask him to return to the ward and apologize to the medical student.

C Apologize on behalf of the registrar, and ask the student not to say anything to anyone else.

D Suggest that the student talk to the firm consultant about the episode.

E Tell the student that they would be less likely to provoke a negative response if their knowledge base was better.

6. You are a lone FY1 doctor seeing a post-operative patient with atrial fibrillation and a heart rate of 160 bpm. Before you finish your assessment, the patient starts to mumble incoherently and will not follow commands or open his eyes.

Choose the THREE most appropriate actions to take in this situation

A Ensure that the patient has a valid Not For Resuscitation order in case they suffer a cardiac arrest.

B Accept that 160 bpm might be normal for this patient.

C Shout for help.

D Ask the nursing staff to put out a peri-arrest call.

E Ensure that you have good intravenous access and give a fluid challenge.

F Ask the patient's family to attend as their relative is probably dying.

G Start chest compressions.

H Ensure that you have adequate airway adjuncts to hand.

7. Your FY1 colleague takes a copy of the operating list home every evening to prepare for the following day in theatre.

Rank in order the following actions in response to this situation (1 = Most appropriate; 5 = Least appropriate)

A Suggest that your colleague makes a simple list of operations to take home.

B Take your own list home so that you can prepare for the theatre list as well.

C Suggest that it is unfair he is 'getting ahead'.

D Speak to the consultant about your colleague's behaviour.

E Inform your colleague that he should not be taking home any list containing confidential patient information.

8. The registrar asks you to teach two medical students who have only just begun their training. You have a long list of jobs to complete and your SHO has just called in sick.

Rank in order the following actions in response to this situation (1 = Most appropriate; 5 = Least appropriate)

A Tell the registrar that you are too busy to look after students.

B Allow the students to shadow you for half an hour, and then ask them to leave.

C Ask the students to attempt to take blood from a few of the patients in exchange for some teaching.

D Allow the students to shadow you completing your routine jobs, before sending them to take a history from a few patients.

E Postpone your ward jobs in order to teach the students for an hour.

9. Your registrar informs you that there is a peritonitic patient intubated on the intensive therapy unit (ITU), waiting to be transferred back to theatre. You have never felt a genuine 'surgical abdomen' before and are keen to utilize this opportunity.

Choose the THREE most appropriate actions to take in this situation

A Do not examine the patient as you have not obtained consent.

B Send a text message to another FY1 doctor to suggest that he examines the patient as well.

C Use this opportunity to read up about causes of a 'surgical abdomen'.

D Examine the patient as this is a valuable learning opportunity.

E Try to contact the patient's next of kin to ask if you can examine the patient.

F Complete your routine ward tasks before going to see the patient.

G Introduce yourself to the ITU consultant and ask if you can examine the patient.

H Go and see the patient, but do not examine their abdomen.

10. You are a new FY1 doctor in surgery and have been asked to see a patient in urinary retention that requires a catheter. You have only ever performed catheterization on a model and are not feeling particularly confident.

Rank in order the following actions in response to this situation (1 = Most appropriate; 5 = Least appropriate)

A Attempt the procedure after talking to the patient, and then ask for help if unsuccessful.

B Call the registrar and ask them to supervise your first catheterization.

C Attempt the procedure without warning the patient about your inexperience.

D Ask another FY1 doctor who is more confident with procedures to help.

E Wait until the end of your shift and then hand the job over to the night team.

11. You are driving home from your evening on call when you remember a chest X-ray that needed to be reviewed for a patient with a newly inserted chest drain. You forgot to hand it over to your colleague who was taking over.

Rank in order the following actions in response to this situation (1 = Most appropriate; 5 = Least appropriate)

A Put the issue out of your mind—it is important to 'turn off' after work.

B Make a note to check the result first thing in the morning before the ward round.

C Drive back to the hospital to check the X-ray yourself.

D Contact the on-call doctor through switchboard and ask them to check the X-ray.

E Reflect about the factors that might have led to forgetting the X-ray.

12. You are working on call covering the medical wards. The registrar asks you to place a chest drain in a patient with a confirmed empyema who is becoming increasingly breathless. As a respiratory FY1 doctor, you have seen many chest tubes being inserted but have yet to place one. The registrar is very busy and will not be able to help.

Choose the THREE most appropriate actions to take in this situation

A Call the registrar and explain that you cannot safely perform the procedure alone but would be grateful if he could supervise you.

B Call the registrar back to say that you are unwilling to do as he asks.

C Use the *Oxford Handbook for the Foundation Programme* to guide your attempt at independently inserting the chest drain.

D Begin to insert the chest drain and contact the on-call registrar if you encounter difficulties.

E Contact your Educational Supervisor at the first possible opportunity to discuss the appropriateness of this request.

F Contact another senior colleague if the on-call registrar does not answer or offers no further support.

G Set up the equipment and explain the procedure to the patient.

H Remind the registrar of the chest drain again in a couple of hours when he is less busy.

13. You are looking after Sally who has become increasingly unwell due to heart failure, despite maximal diuretic therapy. Both you and your registrar believe that Sally would benefit from inotrope therapy on the ITU. The patient's son and the nursing staff feel that aggressive escalation of treatment would not benefit Sally.

Rank in order the following actions in response to this situation (1 = Most appropriate; 5 = Least appropriate)

A Refer Sally to the ITU, as you are ultimately responsible for the patient.

B Read through the medical notes, and try to understand why the family and nursing staff might not want to escalate treatment.

C Tell the patient's brother and nursing staff to think carefully about the options and that you will do as they want if all members agree.

D Document your discussion with the family and stop all active treatment in order to ameliorate the patient's suffering.

E Contact a senior doctor to ask them to make a decision.

14. You are just starting your shift as the evening on-call medical FY1 doctor and have been handed over a long list of jobs, as well as answering bleeps from nursing staff. You need to prioritize tasks.

Rank in order the following in response to this situation (1 = Most appropriate; 5 = Least appropriate)

A An upset patient who wants to discuss her forthcoming endoscopy on the next day.

B An 80-year-old man who has had a fall and hit his head but appears lucid.

C A 70-year-old with a past history of myocardial infarction who has just become unresponsive.

D A 50-year-old man after an elective herniotomy who is still awaiting prescription laxatives and painkillers before he can be discharged.

E A 30-year-old man with renal colic requiring analgesia review for '10/10' pain.

15. You are working as the orthopaedic FY1 doctor when you are called by the orthopaedic registrar on your mobile about a patient who will be arriving on the private ward. He asks you to clerk, cannulate, and initiate intravenous fluids, as the patient will be undergoing elective surgery the following morning.

Rank in order the following actions in response to this situation (1 = Most appropriate; 5 = Least appropriate)

A Prioritize the preoperative clerking and fluid administration alongside your other tasks.

B Contact a responsible person (e.g. duty manager) to ask about the appropriateness of doing jobs on the private ward.

C Suggest that the registrar comes in to complete the clerking if he has agreed to see the consultant's private patient.

D Help if possible, but inform the registrar that this is not a long-term solution for managing private patients.

E Agree to complete the tasks for a reasonable fee.

16. A 40-year-old patient is admitted for an elective procedure on your surgery ward. After reading an article in a newspaper about statins, he tells you he would like them to be prescribed. He is at low risk of cardiovascular disease.

Rank in order the following actions in response to this situation (1 = Most appropriate; 5 = Least appropriate)

A Write a prescription for statins.

B Explain that the high cost of statins means they can only be prescribed to high-risk patients.

C Write to his GP, asking them to discuss the patient's request.

D Inform the patient that he does not have a high enough risk of cardiac disease to gain sufficient benefit from the medication.

E Refer the problem to your consultant.

17. After a ward round, you are approached by one of the patients who says that they are 'scared' and no longer want a bronchoscopy the following day.

Rank in order the following actions in response to this situation (1 = Most appropriate; 5 = Least appropriate)

A Discuss the patient's decision with the nursing staff.

B Explain the benefits of the procedure and insist that she receives it no matter what.

C Explore alternative investigations.

D Establish the patient's concerns.

E Take the patient to see a coronary angiography being performed.

18. You are working in paediatrics and have made two attempts at cannulating a 7-year-old with diabetic ketoacidosis. The mother is becoming quite frustrated and refuses any further attempts.

Choose the THREE most appropriate actions to take in this situation

A Tell the mother that the next attempt will be successful.

B Explain that you will ask a colleague to try if the next attempt fails.

C Encourage oral intake and clearly document that the parent refused cannulation.

D Stop the fluids and resite the cannula if the patient deteriorates.

E Tell the mother that her daughter will probably die without intravenous fluids.

F Document the number of attempts at cannulation afterwards.

G Persist with cannulation attempts, as the mother cannot refuse treatment on her child's behalf.

H Explain carefully why a cannula is necessary.

19. You are an FY1 doctor reviewing patients with your consultant. The consultant tells Doug, a 30-year-old man, that he has a staghorn calculus and must have an operation which will leave a nephrostomy. The consultant leaves once the consent form is signed, but Doug looks as if he still has more questions.

Rank in order the following actions in response to this situation (1 = Most appropriate; 5 = Least appropriate)

A Tell the patient that your consultant will come back later to answer questions.

B Explain that you will come back shortly in case he has any more questions.

C Insist that the consultant stays until he has answered the patient's questions.

D Continue with reviewing patients with the consultant, but see Doug later to answer any questions.

E Let your consultant continue reviewing other patients alone, but remain behind to answer Doug's questions.

20. You have received several complaints from the nursing staff about Michael, who has learning difficulties and has been mobilizing unsafely around the ward. He has become increasingly challenging to manage.

Rank in order the following actions in response to this situation (1 = Most appropriate; 5 = Least appropriate)

A Ask whether a 'special' nurse can be assigned for one-to-one care.

B Attempt to explain to Michael, as far as possible, that it is unsafe for him to move around the ward.

C Suggest distracting interventions.

D Prescribe 'as required' (PRN) sedation.

E Prescribe sedation when Michael becomes particularly agitated and endangers himself or others.

21. Jessie was admitted under the gastroenterology team for chronic abdominal pain. Investigations have not yielded any findings, and your consultant believes that the patient should be discharged with follow-up from the pain team. The patient and her family do not believe she can go home with such severe pain.

Choose the THREE most appropriate actions to take in this situation

A Delete the patient from your list, so that she can remain an inpatient for a few more days.

B Explore Jessie's concerns about going home.

C Promise that you will ensure that the pain team appointment is made within two weeks.

D Tell Jessie the bed is needed for more urgent cases.

E Carefully explain the nature of chronic abdominal pain.

F Ensure that the pain team is involved with discharge planning, so that appropriate analgesia can be provided in the community.

G Prescribe 'as required' (PRN) oral morphine until the patient is discharged.

H Tell Jessie that she needs to learn to accept the pain as it cannot be helped.

22. Six hours ago, you prescribed intravenous antibiotics for a surgical patient for a suspected pelvic abscess. During your afternoon ward round, you find that the antibiotics have still not been given by the nurse.

Rank in order the following actions in response to this situation (1 = Most appropriate; 5 = Least appropriate)

A Contact the pharmacy and seek advice about how to prepare the infusion yourself.

B Inform the Ward Sister that the antibiotics have been dangerously delayed.

C Ensure that the nurse understands the importance of giving antibiotics promptly.

D Approach the nurse on her break, and insist that she prepares the intravenous antibiotics immediately.

E Allow the nurse to complete her jobs without further instruction—she will administer the infusion when she has time.

23. Your SHO prescribes a large dose of gentamicin for a patient with severe renal failure. You notice this when rewriting the drug chart, thankfully before this renotoxic drug was administered. Your SHO thanks you for stopping the prescription in time.

Rank in order the following actions in response to this situation (1 = Most appropriate; 5 = Least appropriate)

A Inform the hospital pharmacy.

B Record a critical incident form for a near miss.

C Inform your consultant at the next available opportunity.

D Do nothing further, as the SHO simply forgot that caution is needed when prescribing gentamicin for patients with renal impairment.

E Note 'renal impairment' somewhere appropriate on the drug chart.

24. While eating lunch in the hospital canteen, you overhear a nurse describing a junior doctor as 'incompetent'. The doctor is readily identifiable, but the nurse seems unaffected by the attention she is attracting from surrounding diners.

Rank in order the following actions in response to this situation (1 = Most appropriate; 5 = Least appropriate)

A Speak to the nurse on the ward later on to explain that such comments in a public environment are unprofessional.

B Let the nurse know that she can be overheard by other diners.

C Speak to someone in the nursing hierarchy to reinforce the message about not publicly undermining colleagues.

D Let the junior doctor concerned know what was said about him.

E Do nothing as this is a public venue and the nurse is on her break.

25. An FY1 colleague who works on your ward consistently struggles to take blood from patients. The samples he has successfully obtained are usually haemolysed.

Rank in order the following actions in response to this situation (1 = Most appropriate; 5 = Least appropriate)

A Ignore the problem, as it is your colleague's concern.

B Email his Clinical Supervisor.

C Contact your consultant immediately to inform him of your colleague's difficulties.

D Help your colleague improve on the ward and by using a skills laboratory if there is one.

E Suggest that your colleague asks a senior for help.

26. You are finding it particularly difficult to work with your new SHO. She is condescending, undermines your management, and has often belittled you in front of senior colleagues.

Choose the THREE most appropriate actions to take in this situation

A Adopt a more subordinate position as her junior colleague.

B Ask your colleagues within the medical team whether they find your SHO difficult to work with.

C Do nothing, provided that her behaviour does not impact on clinical care.

D Ensure that your jobs are done well to avoid avoidable criticism.

E Remind the SHO about your relative inexperience in medicine.

F Speak to a senior colleague for advice.

G Discuss your feelings with the SHO.

H Try to challenge your SHO's clinical knowledge in an effort to impress her.

27. You have just started working on the care of the elderly ward. Despite your relative inexperience, you are certain that your consultant has recklessly discharged unwell patients many times over a four-week period. However, he is well regarded on the ward by patients and nurses. You have never heard another doctor complain about his practice.

Choose the THREE most appropriate actions to take in this situation

A Ask your consultant about specific discharges with which you are unhappy.

B Contact the GMC to raise your concerns.

C Record the events clearly on your medical blog.

D Do nothing as you are alone in thinking that the consultant's decisions are flawed.

E Do nothing as you have no real proof of poor practice.

F Discuss your concerns privately with another senior colleague.

G Contact your Educational Supervisor.

H Inform the Medical Director.

28. You are clerking a young child in the preoperative admissions clinic. You note that the parents are somewhat untidy, with dirty hands and clothes. You consider what to document in the medical notes.

Rank in order the following actions in response to this situation (1 = Most appropriate; 5 = Least appropriate)

A Complete your detailed entry in the notes once you have clerked everyone at the preoperative assessment clinic.

B Briefly summarize your clinical assessment.

C Document the impression that you have formed of the parents' suitability for raising the child.

D Document your detailed physical examination findings of the child.

E Write your notes once your senior colleagues agree with your findings.

29. You have just completed your assessment of a patient who is hypotensive and asked the nurses to administer intravenous fluids. You are bleeped by another ward to say that a patient is pyrexial. While you are taking this call, your crash bleep summons you to a third ward.

Rank in order the following actions in response to this situation (1 = Most appropriate; 5 = Least appropriate)

A Many doctors carry crash bleeps and you should prioritize the patient you are currently treating.

B Attend the crash call, but return later to document your assessment retrospectively.

C Document your current assessment of the patient who is hypotensive and then attend the crash call.

D See the febrile patient after the crash call and then return to document your approach to the hypotensive patient.

E Do not document anything as the unwell patients are a priority.

30. You are being shadowed by a medical student while on call. You receive three bleeps in quick succession: a respiratory patient looking increasingly unwell, blood cultures needed for a febrile patient, and a disgruntled relative wanting to complain about your consultant.

Choose the THREE most appropriate actions to take in this situation

A Ask the medical student to assess the respiratory patient, and you will review shortly afterwards.

B Review the respiratory patient with the medical student.

C Suggest that the student takes blood from the febrile patient.

D Review the respiratory patient alone.

E Do the blood cultures first in case the patient's fever subsides.

F Suggest that the student speaks to the disgruntled relative.

G Meet the relative by yourself on the ward.

H Speak to the relative, together with a nurse, in a side room.

Second exam

1. During your own ward round, you hear a healthcare assistant (HCA) behind a curtain being verbally abusive towards a patient. The patient is disabled and known to have challenging learning disabilities. The patients and staff around the bay do not intervene.

Rank in order the following actions in response to this situation (1 = Most appropriate; 5 = Least appropriate)

A Show your disapproval to the staff in the bay for not responding.

B Contact the Care Quality Commission anonymously to avoid raising the issue with employees of your Trust.

C Ask if other staff have noticed similar behaviour from the HCA.

D Approach the curtain and ask to speak with the HCA.

E Discuss the issue with the nurse in charge (e.g. Matron) upon their arrival.

2. A patient's niece is concerned about the standard of care her relative is receiving and asks you whether she should make a complaint and how to go about doing so.

Rank in order the following actions in response to this situation (1 = Most appropriate; 5 = Least appropriate)

A Establish what she is concerned about and escalate the issues accordingly.

B Direct her to the Patient Advice and Liaison Service (PALS) in case they are able to assist her better.

C Offer to investigate, but explain that a formal complaint is unlikely to resolve matters.

D Agree regarding her assessment, and encourage her to proceed with a formal complaint.

E Notify the Sister in charge that a patient's relative is concerned about standards of care and a complaint may be received in this regard.

3. You review a patient in the Medical Assessment Unit with your SHO, after seeing the patient and clerking them in yourself. The SHO is happy with your entry in the medical notes and agrees to complete a work-based assessment for examining the patient, despite having not seen you examine the patient.

Choose the THREE most appropriate actions to take in this situation

A Tell the SHO that you need more detailed feedback if you are to develop as a doctor.

B Thank the SHO and ask if you could present the case to her later for your own experience.

C Ask the SHO to watch you examine the patient and then complete an assessment.

D Ask the SHO if he will complete two work-based assessments at the same time.

E Examine the patient as formally as possible, even though you are not being assessed.

F Thank the SHO and forward him an electronic form to complete.

G Examine the patient a few hours later when someone might be available to assess you.

H Tell your Educational Supervisor how difficult it is to get senior colleagues to complete formal assessments

4. A patient whom you have looked after for several weeks approaches you and hands you a cheque for a substantial amount. She insists, despite your protests, that you take the gift for all the hard work you have done for her on the ward.

Choose the THREE most appropriate actions to take in this situation

A Take the cheque and then ask an appropriate person within the Trust whether this is allowed.

B Suggest that the patient donates the money to the hospital charity.

C Tell the patient you will only accept half the amount she has offered.

D Covertly return the cheque to the patient's husband on his next hospital visit.

E Ensure the patient has signed a written statement to avoid accusations of criminality.

F Ask the patient to consider her decision very carefully.

G Thank the patient, but politely refuse her offer.

H Refer to a senior in the Trust for advice.

5. An obstetrics and gynaecology audit reveals that your consultant appears to have worse mortality outcomes than the national average. You consider what to do in light of these findings.

Rank in order the following actions in response to this situation (1 = Most appropriate; 5 = Least appropriate)

A Inform the Care Quality Commission about your consultant's mortality figures, as this is an issue of patient safety.

B Email the other consultants for advice about the data.

C Discuss your findings with the consultant alone.

D Submit the audit report without the consultant's data.

E Obtain further patient and perioperative data on the consultant's cases.

6. Your consultant asks you to look after all her patients, including those on the private ward of the hospital. You feel stretched by the additional tasks and regularly leave work after your scheduled hours.

Rank in order the following actions in response to this situation (1 = Most appropriate; 5 = Least appropriate)

A Ignore bleeps from the private ward; if the consultant wants you, he will contact you.

B Arrange a meeting with your consultant to discuss your workload.

C Ask private patients to consider returning to the NHS ward.

D Explain the situation to another consultant.

E Ask the consultant for additional reimbursement in return for providing more of your time for assisting with his private patients.

7. You receive a bleep from your consultant, asking you to consent Mrs Robbins, who is third on today's theatre list for an inguinal hernia repair. You have received teaching from the consultant about the theory of hernias a few months ago, although you have never seen a hernia repair. You also have a mounting list of ward jobs which need to be completed before lunchtime teaching.

Rank in order the following actions in response to this situation (1 = Most appropriate; 5 = Least appropriate)

A Explain to the consultant that you are not able to consent the patient as you do not have the necessary experience.

B Ask the on-call surgical registrar to take the consent.

C Consent the patient immediately.

D Complete your urgent ward jobs before attempting to consent the patient.

E Ask the senior surgical Ward Sister to show you how to consent properly for this operation.

8. Your registrar asks you to book an urgent colonoscopy for one of the ward patients to 'exclude a gastrointestinal bleed'. The patient has not given any symptoms that you feel would indicate this, and you are struggling to articulate a good reason on the request form.

Rank in order the following actions in response to this situation (1 = Most appropriate; 5 = Least appropriate)

A Explain to your consultant you cannot order the colonoscopy as you disagree that it is appropriate.

B Ask your team's SHO whether they can explain why the colonoscopy is necessary.

C Ask the registrar what the scan is for.

D Tell the endoscopist you disagree with doing the scan but have been told that it is urgent.

E Book an abdominal CT scan instead, and later reconsider the colonoscopy based on the results.

9. The overnight on-call SHO identifies an error on your patient's drug chart, in which you have prescribed methotrexate, instead of metronidazole. She has spotted and corrected it before the drug was administered but feels that your Clinical Supervisor should be informed. You feel this is probably due to staff shortages on your ward.

Rank in order the following actions in response to this situation (1 = Most appropriate; 5 = Least appropriate)

A Accept responsibility while explaining factors that contributed to the error.

B Explain to the SHO that this was not your fault because the hospital has failed to staff the ward to safe levels.

C Reflect on the error and its reasons using your e-portfolio to avoid this happening again.

D Ask the SHO not to contact your Clinical Supervisor, as this was an isolated error.

E Ask to meet your Clinical Supervisor to discuss the error and your concerns about staffing levels.

10. The nurse asks you to see a trauma patient who has just become conversant on the ITU ward. He wants to know whether he is likely to be able to walk again, given his pelvic fractures. You are certain that he will be able to walk but are unsure how long he will need to remain on bed rest and do not remember much else about the management of pelvic fractures.

Rank in order the following actions in response to this situation (1 = Most appropriate; 5 = Least appropriate)

A Offer to ask the consultant to come by and answer the patient's questions.

B Go away and read up about the management of pelvic fractures, so you are able to answer these questions.

C Tell the patient that he will be able to walk after sufficient bed rest.

D Explain how most patients with pelvic fractures do recover their mobility after sufficient bed rest, but you will help find out the plan in his case.

E Explain how you are unable to answer complex technical questions, given your junior position within the clinical team.

11. A written complaint is made against you regarding your management of a patient who was readmitted with an obstructed hernia. You had seen the patient and felt that he had a 'benign' abdomen, but had failed to document your findings in any further detail. The patient required emergency surgery to relieve the obstructed and incarcerated hernia upon readmission 24 hours later.

Choose the THREE most appropriate actions to take in this situation

A Record your formal response and inform your defence organization.

B Amend your written entry to honestly reflect the clinical findings that you encountered that led you to believe the patient could be discharged.

C Respond to the complaint at a moment of convenience, as the clinical care of your current patients remains your priority.

D Reflect on the case and what you could do differently to mitigate the risk.

E No further action is required, as it refers to a post that you have now rotated out of.

F Explain the factors, including short staff, long hours, and fatigue, that led to you being unable to complete a thorough clerking of every patient.

G Amend the written notes to include features that might have been present that are likely to absolve the Trust of any possible complaint.

H Give an accurate description of events within the time frame requested.

12. You find yourself having not had a break or eaten anything since starting your Sunday shift five hours ago. You are feeling fatigued and identify that you have begun incorrectly writing a fluid prescription chart. Having corrected your error, you attempt to leave the ward for a break, at which point the nurse in charge asks you to clerk the preoperative elective patient who has come in the day before his surgery.

Choose the THREE most appropriate actions to take in this situation

A Tell the nurse that she should not bother you for such a routine task.

B Ask the nurse to attempt a brief clerking which you will review on your return.

C Suggest to the nurse that preoperative clerkings can be completed by the day team the following day and that this is not a job for the on-call doctor.

D Offer to clerk the patient after your break.

E Briefly 'eyeball' the patient, and if he looks well, go for your break.

F Ask how urgent the clerking is, e.g. any immediate drugs the patient needs prescribing, and then use this to prioritize the task.

G Complete the patient clerking immediately.

H Explain to the Ward Sister that you intended to have a short break.

13. You are working on the gastroenterology ward and have performed several ascitic drain insertions under the supervision of the registrar. Your registrar insists he is confident with your performance and asks you to perform one independently, although you realize you have never actually obtained consent for this procedure.

Rank in order the following actions in response to this situation (1 = Most appropriate; 5 = Least appropriate)

A Obtain verbal consent with the Ward Sister as a witness.

B Seek legal advice prior to beginning the consent process.

C Obtain verbal consent before documenting in the medical notes that 'the patient has been consented' in the notes.

D Decline to perform the procedure, as only registrars and consultants are able to provide consent.

E Complete a formal written consent form.

14. You reach the end of your shift on a general surgery ward and receive a phone call from the nurse coordinator, informing you of a long list of jobs which she insists are completed today. You have consistently finished two hours late every day this week.

Rank in order the following actions in response to this situation (1 = Most appropriate; 5 = Least appropriate)

A Finish for the day and review the tasks in the morning.

B Ask the coordinator to speak with the on-call doctor to review the tasks.

C Ask the coordinator to do what she is able to herself, before contacting the on-call doctor if she feels there is anything else that must be done before tomorrow.

D Assess the jobs and complete as many tasks as possible within the next hour.

E Identify and complete the most urgent tasks before handing over to the on-call doctor.

15. A hip CT scan for an orthopaedic patient demonstrates a small abdominal mass of undetermined significance, and the radiologist recommends repeat imaging at one month.

Rank in order the following actions in response to this situation (1 = Most appropriate; 5 = Least appropriate)

A Ask the patient to inform his GP of the CT finding and the need for further tests, as soon as he is discharged from the hospital.

B Ask a nurse to explain the report findings and follow-up treatment required.

C Highlight on the discharge letter this finding and the requirement for a delayed imaging.

D Contact the patient's GP to inform them of this finding.

E Arrange an orthopaedic follow-up appointment for further management of the abdominal mass.

16. You are bleeped by the hospital's senior Matron regarding the 'code black bed crisis' in the hospital. Having spoken to your consultant, she is now instructing you to discharge three surgical patients immediately. Meanwhile you have been called to see a patient who is unwell on one of the outlying wards.

Rank in order the following actions in response to this situation (1 = Most appropriate; 5 = Least appropriate)

A Phone the registrar and ask if there are any spare doctors to assist with your tasks.

B Sympathize with the severity of the bed crisis, but explain how you have more urgent matters to deal with, and refer her to your registrar.

C Take a few minutes to complete a very brief discharge of the three patients before attending to the care of the unwell patient.

D Ask the Matron to complete the discharge letter, but agree to sign a blank copy in advance to facilitate a fast discharge.

E Agree to complete the discharge letters once you have stabilized your unwell patient.

17. You are sharing ward jobs with another FY1 doctor on a busy medical ward. After quickly dividing the tasks, you later find that your colleague has begun an ascitic drain on the incorrect liver patient.

Choose the THREE most appropriate actions to take in this situation

A Allow your colleague to complete the task, as it risks looking more unprofessional stopping the procedure part way through.

B Tell the FY1 doctor to report himself to the GMC for not confirming the patient's identity.

C Complete a critical incident form.

D Ask the FY1 doctor to stop performing the procedure immediately.

E Allow your colleague to insert the drain, before explaining to the patient that it was in order to obtain an ascitic fluid sample to exclude infection.

F Obtain an abdominal ultrasound to confirm correct drain placement.

G Accept total responsibility for this error.

H Suggest that the FY1 doctor apologizes for the error.

18. A patient's relative asks you to speak with her sister, who is increasingly worried about the Hartmann's procedure and stoma formation planned for her tomorrow.

Choose the THREE most appropriate actions to take in this situation

A Ask the relative to explore any concerns and get back to you if there is anything that you can help with.

B Speak to the family to identify any of the patient's concerns.

C Talk the patient through the procedure and answer any questions she might have.

D Ask the patient to share her concerns.

E Inform the patient that she may risk compromising the safety of other patients if she does not decide whether to go ahead with the surgery.

F Explain to the patient how she should not worry about stomas as they are easily reversed.

G Inform your surgical seniors promptly if the patient appears to show doubt about the procedure.

H Arrange an urgent psychiatry referral.

19. A transplant patient has attended the GP practice at which you are working, having agreed to assist you with the teaching of a group of medical students. Unfortunately, the patient appears particularly distressed, as her husband has recently been admitted to hospital and, despite ten minutes of conversation, remains particularly tearful.

Rank in order the following actions in response to this situation (1 = Most appropriate; 5 = Least appropriate)

A Explore the patient's personal circumstances and current concerns in order to impart valuable lessons in communication skills.

B Provide a lecture-based teaching on transplants.

C Try to ignore the issue, and perform a brief examination of the patient's abdominal system.

D Continue with the bedside teaching as planned, explaining that patients with chronic diseases often become emotional for a variety of reasons.

E Try to provide bedside teaching, but inform the patient that you would be happy to stop if she wishes.

20. A patient is readmitted to the A&E for the fifth time in three months with recurrent leg pains. The patient has been reviewed extensively by numerous medical doctors, emergency doctors, and the patient's GP, but the patient remains anxious about these intermittent attacks. You complete a full work-up and establish no new findings, and in the context of his previous admissions accept that there is nothing more you are able to offer. Your registrar is insistent that you review your patients more expeditiously.

Rank in order the following actions in response to this situation (1 = Most appropriate; 5 = Least appropriate)

A Explore the patient's psychological and social well-being despite prolonging your assessment of the patient.

B Explore whether the patient wishes to consider alternative/complementary therapies.

C Refer the patient to another colleague in the A&E.

D Explain to the patient that you have only a limited time to spend with each patient and that you cannot offer him anything else.

E Refer the patient to a pain specialist.

21. Steven is a 40-year-old paranoid schizophrenic who has returned to your ward with a severe chest infection. You attempt to recommence intravenous antibiotics, as decided by the medical team, but the patient refuses. Steven's mother is distressed at the delay in treatment, stating that 'this happens every time' and gives you permission as his mother to begin treatment.

Rank in order the following actions in response to this situation (1 = Most appropriate; 5 = Least appropriate)

A Defer the decision to a senior colleague.

B Administer the intravenous antibiotics, irrespective of Steven's wishes.

C Ask the mother to help establish whether Steven has capacity to decide for himself.

D Attempt to establish whether Steven lacks capacity by reading through the medical notes.

E Assess Steven's capacity for refusing this treatment.

22. Your consultant asks you to make a patient referral to the drugs and alcohol liaison service in order to arrange methadone replacement for an intravenous drugs user, during the afternoon ward round. The patient already appears to be suffering from withdrawal symptoms. The registrar later informs you that you might spend an hour trying to locate the correct office and arranging the referral, and you should instead defer the referral until tomorrow as there are plenty of more important patients and problems to deal with.

Rank in order the following actions in response to this situation (1 = Most appropriate; 5 = Least appropriate)

A Ask the shadowing student doctor to attempt to locate the office and make the referral, even though referrals are exclusively made by doctors.

B Complete the jobs that your registrar has asked you to do, before attempting to refer the patient to the drug and alcohol service at the end of the day.

C Follow the registrar's instructions and make the referral first thing in the morning.

D Explain the importance of treating withdrawal and suggest that your tasks be reprioritized.

E Issue a formal complaint to your consultant that the registrar is neglecting this patient.

23. A patient appears more confused than you previously recall during your ward round, and you feel this is not in keeping with his previously diagnosed condition.

Choose the THREE most appropriate actions to take in this situation

A Quickly examine the patient, with a view to performing a more detailed review tomorrow.

B Explain to the patient that you will return to review him in more detail after the ward round.

C Consider requesting appropriate investigations.

D Document in the notes that the patient appears more confused, and continue with the ward round.

E Establish his Abbreviated Mental Test Score (AMTS).

F Suggest that the patient be transferred to the psychiatric ward for further assessment of his mental function.

G Perform a full history and examination at a risk of delaying the entire ward round.

H Move on quickly so that you can continue the ward round.

24. A patient attending your GP informs you that he has recently been diagnosed with alcohol-related seizures and has been asked by the hospital doctors to discuss the matter with you in terms of his work. He is a self-employed taxi driver and is the sole provider for his wife and family of three children, and refuses to inform the DVLA.

Choose the THREE most appropriate actions to take in this situation

A Document the advice you have given to the patient.

B Explain the reasonable possibility of another seizure.

C Call the taxi licence issuer to have his taxi licence revoked.

D Agree that he is probably not a danger but that he should inform the DVLA nonetheless.

E Call the DVLA anonymously, but keep this from the patient to maintain his trust.

F Tell the patient that you must inform the taxi licence issuer and call them, even if he refuses consent.

G Inform the patient that you will need to inform the DVLA if he refuses.

H Ask the patient's wife to bring in his driving licence to the practice, so it can be destroyed.

25. A physiotherapist informs you that she has seen a nurse take money from the wallet of a demented patient.

Rank in order the following actions in response to this situation (1 = Most appropriate; 5 = Least appropriate)

A Ask the physiotherapist to establish some more details first by speaking to the patient before making her claim.

B Establish exactly what the physiotherapist saw before informing the Ward Sister.

C Report the incident to your Clinical Supervisor.

D Confront the nurse and ask her to empty her pockets.

E Make a non-urgent phone call to your local police station.

26. Morning handover from night SHOs to junior doctors working during the day appears to be increasingly rushed, and you have noted on several occasions blood tests and investigations not effectively handed over. You feel this may be related to the speed with which the handover takes place, although the registrars and consultants appear to be happy with the pace of the morning handover.

Rank in order the following actions in response to this situation (1 = Most appropriate; 5 = Least appropriate)

A Highlight your concerns if you identify another urgent task that is not handed over, but otherwise do not mention it for fear of causing difficulties.

B Speak with your Clinical Supervisor to explain that handover is inadequate.

C Register formal complaints for those colleagues whom you feel might be responsible for information not being handed over in the past.

D Ensure that your own handover is effective.

E Organize a meeting with the other junior doctors to explain your concerns regarding the efficacy of your handover.

27. Your SHO colleague is going through a separation with his wife and is scheduled to attend numerous civil court hearings over the coming weeks. His performance does not seem to be affected, but you think that he does seem more despondent than usual.

Rank in order the following actions in response to this situation (1 = Most appropriate; 5 = Least appropriate)

A Email your consultant immediately, as you are obliged to ensure patient safety.

B Explore how your colleague is feeling and what kind of support they feel they need.

C Advise your colleague to see a counsellor.

D Continue to observe your colleague's performance at work, but do not mention this matter to anyone else for the moment.

E Advise your colleague to speak to their Educational Supervisor.

28. You are an FY1 doctor working at a GP surgery and seeing 42-year-old Kimberly, who has returned after one week with continuing joint discomfort. At the end of the consultation, she seems relieved, as she found the last internal examination quite uncomfortable and was hoping to avoid another again today. Looking through the computerized notes, you cannot find any note of an internal examination by your FY1 colleague during her last visit and are unsure why this would have been performed.

Choose the THREE most appropriate actions to take in this situation

A Speak to the FY1 doctor during the lunchtime practice meeting.

B Ask the patient to refer herself back to the colleague who performed the examination to seek an explanation.

C Explain to the patient what you think has happened.

D Establish more details about Kimberly's symptoms and what the examination involved.

E Inform the senior GP partner in charge.

F Ask the patient not to disclose anything about the incident to anyone else until your seniors at the practice have discussed the matter with her.

G Approach your FY1 colleague and ask him to describe his review of the patient last week.

H Inform your deanery's training director.

29. You are struggling to schedule an induction meeting with your Clinical Supervisor. Despite this, you feel you have received an adequate induction by the registrars on your firm and feel well supported and able to perform your clinical duties safely. Your supervisor eventually agrees to meet and complete the form between endoscopy cases and only manages to spend a few minutes speaking to you. After completing the online form, he asks you to co-sign the form so the meeting can be officially registered on your e-portfolio.

Choose the THREE most appropriate actions to take in this situation

A Try to identify a more convenient time to sign this form in the near future.

B Report your Clinical Supervisor to the deanery.

C Co-sign the form to confirm that the meeting took place and you have completed your formal Clinical Supervisor meeting.

D Ask your Educational Supervisor to act as your Clinical Supervisor.

E Ask your Clinical Supervisor to arrange for a suitable replacement.

F Refuse to co-sign the form at this moment

G Continue the rotation and persist with similar meetings, accepting that supervisors often have very busy schedules.

H Organize a meeting with the Foundation Programme Director.

30. Ethel is a patient on the orthopaedic ward, making a slow recovery from a neck of femur fracture. At the moment, she is receiving physiotherapy for 15 minutes a day, but you feel that she would benefit from a more intensive regime.

Rank in order the following actions in response to this situation (1 = Most appropriate; 5 = Least appropriate)

A Continue with the current physiotherapy regime.

B Instruct the physiotherapist to double the duration of time spent with Ethel to help expedite her discharge.

C Speak to your orthopaedic seniors and other multi-disciplinary team members to ascertain what they feel about the patient's current physiotherapy regime.

D Invite Ethel and her next of kin to the next multi-disciplinary meeting to raise their concerns at the current level of physiotherapy offered.

E Ask the physiotherapist whether Ethel would benefit from additional physiotherapy input.